BATH BOMBS

Beginner's Guide To Making Amazing Bath Bombs And Bathtub Treats!

Erica Evans

Table of Contents

Lavender and bergamot bath bomb
Lemon and rosemary bath bomb
Sage, mint and tea tree oil bath bombs
Lavender, geranium and rose oil bath bombs
Cedarwood, lemon, clove and orange essential oil bath bomb
Sage and lavender surprise
Gold, myrrh and frankincense bath bombs
Green tea bath bomb
Grapefruit bath bomb
Honey and milk heart treats
Aloe bubble bath bomb
Oatmeal bath bomb
Blueberry bath bomb recipe
Apricot bath bombs
White tree coconut oil bath bomb
Ginger peach bath bomb
Salty caramel bath bombs
Rose and bergamot bath bomb
Strawberry Shake bath bomb
Cotton Candy bath bomb
Freshly ground coffee bath bombs
Black cherry bath bombs
Green apple bath bomb
Orange dreamsickle bath bomb
Wild bath bomb
Sinus relief bath bomb
Gingersnap cookies bath bombs
Pink salt bath bombs
Jasmine bath bomb
Lemongrass and eucalyptus bath bomb
Lavender and marjoram bath bomb
Orange and vanilla bath bomb
Rose and milk bath bomb

Conclusion

Introduction

How would you feel about sitting in a warm bathtub at the end of hard day's work? Will you not find it extremely relaxing to cool yourself down on a hot summer evening by standing under a cold shower? I bet your mind has already travelled to either one of these situations!

Be it a hot one or a cold one, a bath tends to lend an extremely therapeutic experience to the bather.

Baths help relax a person's mind and body and allow them to stave off stress. A long bath also has proven physical benefits, which makes shower time a true winner.

However, with hectic lives to lead, it becomes all the more difficult for people to make time for long baths. Most people rush in and rush out, and hardly spend any time scrubbing their bodies, while simply focusing on getting soap off of their skin.

That, however, can be changed for good, once you start looking at your bath time as a time to relax and recoil.

What's more, you can make use of bath bombs to enhance your experience and heighten the therapeutic value.

In this book, we will look at bath bombs in detail, encompassing its meaning, history, recipes, precautions etc.

This book is meant to be your comprehensive bath bomb guide and will supply you with all that you need to know about preparing these bombs by your-self.

Chapter 1: Bath Bombs-What Are They?

Since time immemorial, man has taken bath to cleanse his body and remain healthy physically. However, this is not the only purpose that baths can serve.

In this day and age, where everybody leads a stressful life, it becomes all the more important to create a routine that can help reel in a sense of calm relaxation. One such routine can be that of taking long baths. Long baths have the tendency of helping you rewind and relax your mind. You can do away with unnecessary stress and improve your overall level of well being.

Now what if I said it is possible for you to make your long bath even more relaxing? Yes, by making use of bath bombs, you can improve your overall bathing experience and also your mindset. You will feel calmer and far more relaxed owing to the effects of the bomb on your mind and body.

What are bath bombs?

I want you to think back a little and visualize tiny glass jars that were kept on the windowsill by your mother or grandmother. These contained tiny round colored balls. These balls were nothing but bath bombs!

Bath bombs are tiny soap like balls that are used to add to bath water. They contain skin friendly ingredients which can help soften and condition skin, as also promote heady fragrances, which can leave you feeling great about yourself.

These bath bombs are generally made of baking soda and citric acid, both of which react to create an effervescent reaction in the water. They can also produce a sound, which gives them their name.

These bath bombs are generally meant to be used by children to make bath time fun but given their skin conditioning qualities; adults too can make use of these.

These bath bombs are all hand made as it takes careful handling to pack them into small balls or squares. This makes them ideal to be made within the confines of your home.

History of bath bombs

As mentioned earlier, bath time is usually seen as a time to cleanse our bodies. However, it can be much more than just that. You can treat it as a time to relax and recoil and get over your daily stress.

It need not be all serious all the time and you can have fun while having your daily bath.

Before there were bath bombs, there was aromatherapy. Aromatherapy is a concept that revolves around using aromas to help calm down and relax your mind. It calls for the use of different essential oils, each of which has a different effect on your mind and body.

These essential oils are all natural and derived from nature. Invented in 1937 by René-Maurice Gattefosse, these oils were discovered by accident. After burning his hand in the lab, Rene decided to cool it off by pacing his hand in lavender oil instead of water and that's where he discovered the true use of the oil. His hand rapidly healed and he could no longer feel a burning sensation. That is when he decided to experiment with other oils and write down each of their true effects on skin and mind.

In 1989, Mo Constantine is said to have created the first bath bomb. The owner of Lush Cosmetics, a company that is now famous for their bath bombs, is said to have stumbled upon the recipe and decided to open a company to sell the same.

Ever since, bath bombs have become somewhat of a rage and more and more people now use it during bath time. These bath bombs are nothing but soluble soap without any harsh chemicals and unnatural colors.

Bath bombs are named so owing to the way they react with water. The citric acid and sodium bicarbonate react with each other to create an effervescence, which makes it look like a bomb exploding.

Once they dissolve, they make the bath water both colorful and fill in with skin friendly ingredients.

Although most people prefer to buy bath bombs commercially, one can easily make them at home. All you need is a few ingredients that are available to you at home, put them together and create these bombs. You can get your children involved as well and make it a fun and relaxing activity.

In this book, we will look at the different aspects of bath bombs and everything you need to know before getting started with it. It will also provide you with different recipes that you can use to make these bombs.

Let's go!

Chapter 2: Bath Bomb Uses

In the previous chapter, we looked at the basics and history of bath bomb. Let us now look at some of the basic uses of bath bombs and how you can use them.

Skin conditioning

You can use bath bombs to condition and soften your skin. If you have rough skin, then use a bomb that contains vitamin E oil, which can help you soften your skin to a large extent. It will also help in firming up loose skin and get rid of stretch marks. You can also use something containing coconut oil, as it is known to replenish moisture. If you have oily skin then use something containing tea tree oil, as it will help in drawing out excess oil from your skin and can also aid in reducing the occurrence of pimples.

Hair conditioning

You can also use bath bombs while washing your hair. It can contain hair friendly ingredients that will leave your hair feeling soft and shiny. Make use of oils such as rosemary and thyme, which are proven to have hair friendly benefits. Tea tree oil can be used to treat dandruff and improve the quality of your scalp. Using bath bombs containing lavender will leave behind a fun and floral smell, which can help your hair remain fresh and fragrant all through the day!

Stress relief

You can make use of bath bombs to avail relief from stress and anxiety. Bath bombs are great for those that have a hectic lifestyle and need something to cut down on the stress and tension. Bath bombs will leave behind a fun fragrance that will help you diminish your stress. Rose, cedar, geranium, vanilla, orange, cherry blossom etc. are all fragrances that are known to help with stress and can be used to reduce the occurrence of tension and anxiety. In fact, stress relief is the main function of bath bombs and just placing them in the bathroom can help you feel calm and relaxed.

Cold relief

You can make use of bath bombs to avail relief from sinus issues. Use the ones that contain eucalyptus oil as that can help in draining the sinus. You can also use the one containing clove oil. Just add them to your bath and you will see how your sinus is melting away. You need not add a huge quantity and just a small amount can go a long way in helping you avail relief from your cold. In fact, you can use it on a daily basis to stave off the occurrence of cold and cough.

Sprains

Many people suffer from sprains and ligament issues, especially if they are physically active. But there is a solution to this that can provide you with instant relief. You can make use of bath bombs containing peppermint, ginger and rosemary. All of these have proven benefits on helping you relax and heal your muscles. You get rid of sprains, strains and spasms. Just add a bomb or two to the water that you will be using to bathe with. If you want a more concentrated concoction then consider adding two to a bucket of water before lowering the body part with the sprain. This will help you avail quick and lasting relief.

Aromatherapy

Aromatherapy is now considered a bona fide science. It is one where you make use of different aromas to heal yourself mentally and physically. There are many smells to choose from and each one will have a different bearing on your senses. Some of the most preferred smells include rose, lemon, jasmine, lavender, peppermint etc. You can pick the one that you think will work best on your senses and use it to add to your bath bombs. Use these bombs regularly and heighten your bathing pleasure.

Room freshener

If you want a quick solution to refresh your room then you can place a few bath bombs in a bowl and place the bowl under a ceiling fan. You can also place it in front of an air blower, which can help in dissipating the smell of the bath bomb. You can consider crushing some and adding to a bowl of pot Pourri. The Pourri will quickly absorb the smell and refresh your room.

Drawer freshener

Many people complain of a bad odor that can emanate from their closets and drawers. This is especially true with shoe cupboards and so, the best solution is to place a few bath bombs in it to get rid of the smells. You can place them randomly or in a bowl. The bath bombs will help in enlivening the atmosphere inside your cupboard and make it smell amazing. Pick the ones that have a strong smell like bay leaf oil. This will also deter unwanted pests such as cockroaches and silver fish from entering your cupboard and ruining your clothes, shoes and other belongings.

Cleaners

You can make bath bombs that can be used to clean the house. For example, you can make one that contains eucalyptus oil to clean the floor, as it will both lend a sheen to the floor and aid in cutting down on mosquito infestations. Similarly, you can use a bomb containing lavender to get rid of any musty smell from your carpets. You can make bombs depending on what you think will work well. You can look up the oil's properties and then zero in on it. But first test it out on a small patch before using it on a larger area. This is especially important if you have expensive furniture. If the small area does not react adversely to the bath bomb mixture then you can go ahead and use it on the larger surface.

For pets

You can make bath bombs specific to pets. These bombs can contain clove oil, which is great to get rid of ticks, fleas etc. Adding in some vitamin e oil can help soften their coats as well. But make sure you test the product out on a small area before giving your pet a full-fledged bath. Some cats can be extremely sensitive and you must first ask the vet about it before using the bombs.

As you can see, there are many things that you can do with your bath bombs and need not be limited to just a few uses. In fact, you can go ahead and find other uses as well and use these bombs to their full potential.

Chapter 3: Bath Bomb - Basic Recipe

When it comes to making bath bombs at home, it can be quite a simple procedure. There is not too much science involved and you need not get your thinking caps on.

A very basic reaction takes place when your bath bomb hits the water. It contains citric acid crystals and sodium bi carbonate, which create effervescence when they react together.

Citric acid is a mild variety of acid and sodium bi carbonate is a base. The two react and a fizz is created. In fact, it is the same reaction that takes pace when you add Alka Seltzer tablets to water. They too contain pretty much the same ingredients and generate a fizz when they hit water.

The carbon di oxide in it escapes, thereby creating the bubbles in the bath water. This is what makes bath bombs so much fun and interesting for both kids and adults.

Another prominent ingredient that is used is cornstarch. Cornstarch is used as a neutral agent that will help in holding the bomb together. It will not react in any way and only aid in adding volume to the bomb.

Water is added in to bath bomb mixes to help it combine well. You might otherwise find it tough to keep your bath bomb together if you don't add in the water. This might seem strange as the bomb might immediately react with it. However, you need not worry as only a little water will be added in, which will not be sufficient for the bomb to react with. You have to be a little careful though and make use of proper measurements when making these bombs.

Vitamin E oil has several skin benefits, which makes it a great ingredient to add to bath bombs. Vitamin E oil will nourish your skin from the inside out and also has great hair care benefits. You can add just a little, which will suffice for your entire body. It is full of anti-oxidants, which is a primary requirement for healthy, glowing skin.

Vegetable or sunflower oil is used as carrier oils. Both of them will help dissolve the vitamin and essential oils so that it is evenly distributed within the bath bombs. If you try making them without these oils then it will not dissipate easily. You can use any carrier oil you like as long as it has a neutral smell and will not adversely react with the rest of the ingredients. Olive oil will make for great carrier oil, as it will also add in skin and hair benefits. Distilled almond oil also works well.

The bath salts are meant to help your bath bomb turn into a good scrub. A scrub basically aids in removing the dried and dead skin on your body. You can choose Epsom salts or even regular sea salt. Rub the sea salt with a little essential oil to make it a bit more pliable. You can add a quantity that you think will work best to make the bath bomb mixture of a proper consistency.

Food coloring is used to add to bath bombs to make them colorful and interesting. As you know, these bombs are generally aimed at children, who will appreciate the bomb's contribution towards making bath time fun. You can use any color of your choice but ensure that they are food grade. Many people think these can stain the skin and leave behind marks. This is true if you use low quality colors. Buy them from trusted shops. If you don't wish to take a chance then you can skip adding in color to your bath bombs. Colorless ones will still produce effervescence and make it interesting for you.

Essential oils are added in for aroma. You can choose an essential oil that you think works well with your bath bomb. Adding something therapeutic is always recommended. Go for mild ones like rose and lavender when preparing bombs for children and stronger ones like bergamot and peppermint when making it for adults. We have dedicated an entire chapter to essential oils to make it easier for you to pick.

Witch hazel is a spray that you can use to prevent air bubbles from appearing on the bath bomb. They will also hold better if you spray a little on them. However, this is an optional step that you can avoid if you don't have witch hazel with you.

Remember, the fresher the bath bomb, the frizzier it will be. If you allow it to stay too long then it will lose some of its effervescent qualities.

Here is a basic recipe that you need to know when you wish to create bath bombs.

Ingredients:

- Citric acid crystals
- Baking soda
- Cornstarch
- Water
- Vitamin e oil
- Sunflower oil
- Bath salts
- Essential oils
- Food coloring
- Witch hazel (optional)

Method:

You must combine all the wet ingredients in a bowl and set it aside. Add the citric acid and baking soda to a bowl and mix well. Combine the wet with the dry ingredients and make small balls out of it. These need to rest in molds over night before you can use them.

You can spray some witch hazel on them to prevent air bubbles from appearing and also prevent it from breaking.

You can make use of any salts that you think will work well on your skin.

Chapter 4: Bath Bomb Essential Oils

As you know, essential oils are a big part of bath bombs. You cannot make bath bombs without these oils, as that will defeat the purpose. You have to pick essential oils that will leave you feeling amazing about your body and heighten your senses. Here are some essential oils to consider using for making your bath bombs.

Eucalyptus

The first essential oil that we will look at is eucalyptus. This oil is derived from the leaves and bark of the eucalyptus tree. The oil is extremely fragrant and can leave behind a heady feeling. It is possibly the strongest of essential oils and so, should be used with caution. Eucalyptus is used for many purposes. It is used to relive sinus and cold and can also be used to treat mild fever. Adding a few drops to warm water and inhaling the steam can reduce congestion. Eucalyptus also has several skin care benefits such as removing bacteria and reducing the spread of virus. Using a little to dab on pulse points can help in relieving stress and tension as well as inducing a sense of calm and relaxation. Eucalyptus can also successfully keep bugs at bay.

Peppermint

Peppermint can be just as strong as eucalyptus and what many use to create a strong bath bomb. Peppermint will leave your skin tingling. It is known to improve blood circulation and will allow you to maintain healthy, glowing skin. Peppermint is unique oil, which will dominate over the others. So you have to get your combinations right in order to prevent it from taking over your bath bomb's predominant smell. This oil is mainly used during summers, as it will cool your skin down and also has anti-inflammatory properties that will prevent eruptions on your skin.

Ylang-Ylang

Ylang-Ylang is an essential oil that is mostly used in spas, as it will instantly aid in bringing down a person's stress levels. In fact, ylang-ylang has the capacity to reduce heart palpitations. Ylang-ylang is known to promote the release of endorphins. These can aid in pain relief as also help in healing the body from the inside out. Ylang-Ylang also acts as an aphrodisiac. This oil easily blends in with other oils and you don't have to worry about it dominating the others.

Rose

Rose is great for people that want a mild yet soothing fragrance. In fact, rose is a very romantic fragrance that will induce a nice feeling. Rose essential oil is effective as a sleep inducer and having a night bath using rose bath bomb can help you sleep well. Rose can be used as a base note with pretty much any other essential oil of your choice.

Lavender

Lavender is extremely common and one of the most widely used essential oils in the world. Lavender has a very soothing scent that is capable of inducing a very relaxed feeling. Adding just a couple of drops is enough to make your bath bomb smell extremely fragrant. Lavender also has skin care benefits. It will help your skin turn soft, supple and hydrated. Lavender can be used in combination with any other essential oil, as it will lend it a soothing fragrance.

Lemon

Lemon is a great fragrance to add to your bath bombs. A lemony scent is sure to get you in the right mood for a bath. You can add in just a few drops to make your bath bomb extremely fragrant. Lemon can be a stand-alone smell or can be mixed with something fruity such as vanilla. Lemon and orange are both great and will especially be loved by children. However, be a little careful with these as too much can make your bombs smell like dish liquid.

Vanilla

Vanilla is a very basic yet loved fragrance. A simple vanilla flavored bath bomb can be quite an amazing addition to your collection of bath bombs. Drop in one to heighten your senses and treat yourself to a heady fragrance. Vanilla oil can be hard to find but you can make use of vanilla extract or essence instead. Either will lend your bath bomb the ideal fragrance. But you might have to use the extract sparingly as it can be a bit too strong.

Sandalwood

Sandalwood oil is extracted from sandalwood trees. Sandalwood oil is quite rare and also pretty expensive. The oil has a royal fragrance and sure to make your bath time a regal experience. Sandalwood oil is great for skin and can leave it feeling soft, supple and glowing. Sandalwood oil is generally used as stand-alone oil as adding in anything else can eat away into its real fragrance.

Tea tree

Tea tree oil is generally added in with the other oils to make the bath bomb carry an antiseptic quality. Tea tree oil is great for both skin and hair. It has anti-bacterial, anti-viral and anti-inflammatory properties, thereby making it a great product to add to bath bombs. It will help in healing cuts and wounds, prevent any infections, reduce dandruff and promote a healthy scalp. Just a few drops will be enough to help you avail all these benefits and more!

Geranium

Geranium is derived from the flowers and stems of the geranium plant and is a great essential oil to use for your bath bombs. The oil has the capacity to both repair skin and eliminate wrinkles. It will also leave behind a gentle glow. Geranium oil also assists in blood circulation, which makes it an essential ingredient to add to your bath bombs. Geranium has a great fragrance by itself but can be used in combination of others as well.

These form the different essential oils that you can consider for your bath bombs. They can be bought online or specialty stores. However, the best option would be to make them at home using quality, raw materials. This aspect will be dealt with in detail in the next chapter.

Chapter 5: DIY Essential Oils

Essential oils need not always be bought and can be easily made at home. You can make use of the best raw materials to extract the oil. In this chapter, we will look at the procedure that you can adopt to make this oil at home.

Commercially purchased essential oils can be expensive and might contain chemicals that can harm your skin. Homemade ones will be both cheap and contain ingredients that you would source by yourself.

There are many techniques to extract essential oils but we will look at three of the easiest ones that you can use.

For the first one, you will need an extractor machine known as the Distiller. Distillers are easily available and sold widely on online sites. They can be made of steel or any other metal and come in different sizes. But these ready-made ones can be a bit expensive and instead, you can make one by yourself. Here is how to make your own distiller and use it to extract the essential oils.

What you need

- Pressure cooker (buy online)
- Steel tube
- Plastic tube
- Sealant
- Large tub
- Cold water, ice water
- Beaker
- Raw materials for the extraction
- Sterilized glass bottles

Procedure

- Start by cleaning the cooker thoroughly.
- Now take the lid and seal off the steam inducer that is present on it.
- Place the steel tube over the steam outlet and seal it in place with the sealant. Ensure that there is absolutely no gap to allow the steam to escape.
- Now attach the plastic tube to the other end of the steel tube.
- The plastic tube can be coiled a few times.
- Place the coiled tube in the large tub containing the cold water.
- Place the cooker on the heat and fill it up with the raw materials.
- Add in enough water to completely immerse the raw materials.
- Now close the lid tightly and wait for the water to boil.
- Once it does, it will start producing steam.

- This steam will have the essential oil dissolved within in.
- When the hot steam passes through the cold tube, it condenses and the water is collected in the beaker at the end.
- You can wait a while before using a dropper to pick up the oil from the beaker and transferring it into the sterilized bottles.
- Place the bottles in a dark place for 24 hours.
- Your essential oil is now ready to use.
- You can vary the level of concentration by adding less or more raw materials. But this technique is the best one to employ if you wish to extract pure essential oil.

Carrier Oil method

The carrier oil method is one where you make use of a carrier oil to create the essential oil. The carrier oil has to be neutral oil that will not easily mix with the essential oil. The carrier oil can be sunflower oil, olive oil etc. Place the oil in a saucepan. Now add in the raw materials to it and heat it lightly. Once it heats, the raw materials will start mixing in with the oil and release their flavor. Once done, you can distil the carrier oil and store it in storage bottles. It will take some time for the oils to amalgamate and you might have to wait a couple of days for it. This method will not give you the same results as the previous one and the essential oil will not be as strong.

Boiling method

You can boil the raw materials in water and allow them to infuse their flavor into it. This is also not a popular technique and you will be left with a mediocre product. However, it is fine to use it if you are in a hurry. The technique calls for the boiling of the raw materials in distilled water and then straining it to do away with the raw materials. The water then needs to be cooled and you will find the oil on top, which can be extracted. You can also use the cool water to flavor your bath bombs. The essential oil extracted through this technique will not be as strong as the ones that the previous two methods will put out.

Storage

- You can store your essential oil in sterilized glass bottles in a dark environment. This will help them age and develop a strong fragrance. Do not use plastic bottles as they can adversely react with the oils and create an unpleasant odor.

- You have to keep them as away from sunlight as possible as that can tamper with their essential quality.

- You have to make use of labels to mark off these bottles. Apart from writing the name, you must also write down the date of making the oil and also the expiry date. Most essential oils expire in 6 months' time and so, you have to try and use it up within that time.

- Don't mix two or more essential oils in advance. They might react adversely and leave behind an unpleasant odor. It is best to mix them just before using them.

Chapter 6: What To Add To Your Bath Bombs

You need not make your bath bombs out of the basic ingredients alone and make use of some exotic ones as well. Here are the different ones that you can use.

Salts

Salts are great to add to your bath bombs. These slats will not only scrub away dead skin and cells but also nourish your skin in a unique way. They will help in opening up the pores thereby encouraging the absorption of the skin friendly nutrients. Adding in even a small amount of these salts can help you give your skin the much needed boost. You can choose Epsom salt or regular sea salt that has been brushed with some essential oil. Either can go into your bath bomb to make it richer and bulkier. However, you might have to look out for extra sharp particles. Run your hand through the salt first to see if there are any sharp elements within it. Remove and discard them to make the salt ideal to be added to your bath bombs. You can also use refined salt if you think it is a better option.

Sand

If you don't want to use any kind of salt to make your bath bomb, then you can replace it with some sand. Sand can act as an exfoliator and help scrub away all that excess dead skin cells. You can buy sand from a specialty store or pick some up from the beach. You can then sieve it and boil it to remove any impurities. Your sand will then be ready to be added to your bath bomb. Add in just a small amount to see how the bath bomb holds up. If it is too grainy then soften it with some witch hazel before adding to the bomb.

Herbs

You can add in dried or fresh herbs to your bath bomb. Either will work well in creating a unique bath bomb. Dried herbs can include rosemary, thyme and mint. You can dry them out in the sun for some time or use a dehydrator to draw out the moisture content. You can then add them to the bath bomb to enhance their flavor and heighten their effects. Adding in fresh herbs is also an option but that will reduce the shelf life of your bath bomb.

Flowers

You can dry flowers in the sun as well to be added to your bath bombs. If you wish to use the dehydrator then you must ensure that it does not such away the essence of the flowers. You can choose lavender rose, lilies, marigolds etc. Anything that you think will work well with your bath bomb can be dried and added to it. You can keep the bath bomb completely white and add in these colored flowers for an interesting kaleidoscope effect. These will also enhance the skin value of the bath bomb.

Spices

As interesting as it sounds, you can make use of spices to add to your bath bombs as well. Yes, that's right, you can use spices such as clove and cinnamon to be added to your bath bombs. These will not impart their unique flavor but also make the bomb a bit more skin friendly. They will act as an exfoliator and leave behind a heady fragrance. You can either incorporate them within the bomb or pierce them into the bath bomb to help it stay in place. A good tip is to first dry roast the spices to help them release their flavor better before incorporating them in your bath bombs.

Lye

Lye is used to make soap. If you are keen on making a bath bomb cum soap, then you can consider making use of lye. Better known as Sodium laureth sulfate, lye is what gives soap the tendency of becoming frothy. Adding in this chemical will allow you to create a bath bomb that is capable of both acting as a fizzing agent as well as one that will cleanse your skin thoroughly. But be very, very careful, as lye is extremely caustic. You have to wear gloves at all times and ensure that no one is around.

Stems

Stems are great additions to bath bombs. Not many realize that the true flavor of an ingredient lies within its stems. These stems can belong to trees, leaves, flowers etc. For example, the stems of mint leaves will produce a stronger flavor as compared to the leaves themselves. So, you can cut them into small bits and add to your bath bombs. You can dehydrate them or place them under sun for 24 hours. You can also puree them and add to the bath bomb but then again, doing so will reduce their shelf life.

Peels

Lemon, orange and other such citrus fruits carry amazing fragrances within their peels. So, you can remove, dry and use them to make your bath bombs. You can crush them into small pieces and add to the bombs. They will ooze out natural oils, which will make your bombs richer. You can use the different ones all together if you wish to remain with a strong fragrance. When the bath bomb explodes and these peels hit the water, the aroma will fill up the room and heighten your senses.

Glitter

It is a good idea for you to make use of glitter to make your bath bombs fun. Food grade glitter can be used within the bomb or it can be dipped in a bowl containing the glitter. Either way, incorporating it will help you add a whole new dimension to the bath bomb. There are also cosmetic glitters available, which can be added to the bomb. These will leave behind a unique shimmer on your skin. You can use colorful glitter while making bombs for your children and golden for yourself.

Toys

You can also incorporate toys within your bath bombs to make bath times extra fun. These can be miniature toys that can be placed within the bombs so that they will make your children happy. But make sure they are not sharp and are age appropriate. You must keep an eye on your child when they use these bombs. You can also add other things like seashells, mini stars etc.

Do not limit yourself to just these and add in whatever you think will enrich your bath bombs. As long as they will not mingle with the basic composition of a bath bomb, you can add in whatever you think will make them unique and special.

Chapter 7: Bath Bomb Packing And Care

When it comes to packing your bath bombs for storage, you have to keep in mind certain important pointers that are as follows.

Wrap it

Wrapping up your bath bombs is the best way to keep them safe for long. You can make use of cling film to wrap them and store them, as you like. You can also use bubble wrap if you wish to transport them. Be extremely careful while wrapping as these bombs can be delicate and crumble easily. Don't be careless with them once they are wrapped and try to handle them with as much care as possible. A good technique is to cut out sheets of appropriate sizes to wrap the balls without hassle. You don't have to secure it with anything unless it is being transported. In that case, you can make use of tape to hold it in place.

Box it

The best way to preserve your bath bombs is by placing them in boxes. The boxes can be made of wood or metal. Glass jars are also typically used to store these bombs but care must be taken not to use wet hands while reaching for these bombs. You can decorate the boxes and give them away as gifts as well. Try to use big boxes that will hold the bombs in place. At the same time, don't leave too much space as they can move around and might end up breaking. Place a tag on each box to know what lies within it.

Stack it

You can stack the bath bombs on top of each other and create a pyramid. But take care as to not knock them over. This will make it look extremely interesting. You must ask your child to always pick up the one from top and not disturb the bottom as that might knock the structure over. You must individually wrap them with the cling film first and then stack them. Try placing bigger bombs at the bottom and smaller ones on top. You must steady the structure as much as possible before building up on it.

Stand it

You can make use of a cake stand to place your bath bombs. This is a very interesting idea and will make your children happy. You can place the stand in their room or in the bathroom. A cake stand can hold several bath bombs at once. You have to find the space for them and place them in a neat manner. The cake stand can have 2 or more layers and you can fill each one up with bombs of different colors.

Hang it

It is also a great idea for you to hang the bath bombs in your bathroom. You can make use of cling film to wrap the bath bombs and then use twine to further wrap it. This twine can then be suspended from a hanger. You can place the hanger in the bathroom. If you are up for it then you can wrap a wire around the mouth of the Mason jar and suspend it from top. Place the bath bomb within the jar and you can reach into it to pick one up during bath time.

Moisture

You have to ensure that your bath bombs are kept as away from moisture as possible. If moisture hits the bombs, then they will immediately start to crumble, due to the chemical reaction taking place. You have to wrap it up firmly using the cling film to ensure that all moisture is kept out. If you live in humid areas, you can place the bath bombs next to a de-humidifier so that it can prevent the moisture from getting to the bombs. You can also place silica gel pouches within it to help draw out the moisture and keep your bath bombs safe.

Heat

Heat can also negatively impact your bath bombs. You have to keep them as away from a heat source as possible to ensure that they are neatly stacked in a box. Don't handle them in the kitchen or near a heat source. When packing them, take them to a cool area. Avoid taking them under sunlight as well as that will also cause them to melt. Make use of an ice pack to keep them cool if you live in a very hot area. You can also consider placing them in the fridge to help them hold form.

Light

You must also protect them from light sources. Light can cause them to discolor. Try to place them in dark corners. If you have a bright windowsill in your bathroom then consider placing them away from it. You can otherwise place the bath bombs in a dark box to prevent any light from filtering through. Or you can insert a dark cloth inside the jar to keep light from hitting the bath bombs.

Chemicals

Certain chemicals can also adversely react with bath bombs and you must keep them away from it. These chemicals can be quite harsh and damage your bath bombs. The likes of phenols and other floor cleaners might also end up transferring their smells to the bombs, which can make it a bit dangerous. So place them as away from these as possible in order to keep them safe.

Plastics

Certain bath bombs can also adversely react with plastics. So, you must store them in wooden or glass containers that will remain neutral. If you wish to use plastic ones then ensure that the bath bombs are first wrapped tightly with the cling film before being placed within the boxes.

These form the different aspects to bear in mind while taking care of your bath bombs. You have to take good care of them considering the effort that you will put in towards making them.

Chapter 8: Bath Bomb Mistakes To Look Out For

When it comes to making bath bombs, you need to be on the look put for certain mistakes that need to be avoided.

Crumbling

The first mishap to look into is crumbling or cracking bath bombs. Bath bombs can be quite delicate and easily crack or crumble. This mainly happens if the mixture that you have used for the bomb is too dry. It is obvious that a dry mixture will crumble and fall apart. The best solution is to make use of witch hazel or essential oils to keep it altogether. Be careful so as to not pack the bath bombs too tightly. You will end up crumbling them or making them too loose. Try wearing rubber gloves to help them stay together while binding them. Using plastic gloves might make them slip. If you are using bear hands then you can use a little vegetable oil to coat your hands. But don't use too much as that might make the mixture too wet.

Softening

Using too much moisture for your bath bomb will result in a soft mixture that will not hold form. You have to use just the right amount to ensure that the bomb is stable. You can consider using measuring jars and spoons to get the right amount in. The moisture content will vary depending on the ingredients that have gone into the mixture. You can add in a little more cornstarch to balance out the moisture. But remember, you will have to add back in a little of everything to make the bombs maintain their original flavor and texture. So, be careful while adding the water to it lest you end up adding in too much.

Lumps and bumps

Many reasons can result in a lumpy or bumpy bath bomb. You have to ensure that the baking soda that is going in is free from these bumps and lumps. You can consider sieving it first to get rid of any such lumps and bumps. Another reason could be the clumping together of the ingredients with the oil. You have to be a little careful while adding the ingredients to the mixture. If you add in too much at once then you will not be able to take out some of it. Use appropriate spoons and measuring cups to ensure that the right amount goes in. Mix the mixture swiftly once the oil goes in to ensure that no lumps are formed.

Lack of fizz

If there is a lack of fizz in your bath bombs then it means that there is a lack of citric acid in it. You have to increase its content in order to ensure that your bath bomb fizzes. There will be set, pre-determined measurements that you will have to bear in mind while making these bath bombs. You have to maintain the same to ensure that you end up with the right product every time. If your bath bomb still fails to fizz then try reducing the moisture content in it. That will help you increase the fizz.

Expansion

If you spot the bath bomb expanding and overflowing from the mold then it means there is too much moisture within the bath bomb or in the atmosphere. Both will cause the chemical reaction to take place thereby enabling the bomb to expand. You have to make sure that the moisture content in it is not too much and you have not exposed it to the atmosphere. Quickly cover it with cling film to cut out the moisture and see if that works, if it doesn't, then remove the bomb out and rework it.

Discoloration

Discoloration can sometimes happen when you expose the bomb to air. This is predominantly because of air molecules reacting with the bomb and causing it to lose color. If you don't want yours to lose its original color then you will have to be a little generous with your food coloring. Only then will it hold its true color. Discoloration can also occur due to excess moisture, which will start the chemical reaction and cause the bath bomb to lose its color. You have to ensure that there is just enough moisture and cover the bomb to prevent exposure to air.

Shapeless bomb

A shapeless bomb might occur if it is too dry or too moist. It will not fit in well into the mold and you will remain with something that has no proper shape. The best solution to this is to check both these aspects and fix them. If it still remains shapeless then simply roll them into balls and work on another batch to be added to the mold. You can also make use of cookie cutters in place of molds to create the bath bomb shapes. Applying a little oil inside the mold will help you dislodge it with ease.

Witch hazel

If you dint have witch hazel then don't worry, you can use substitutes for it. You can add a little rubbing alcohol to a spray bottle and use it in place of the witch hazel. It will serve the same purpose and you can eliminate any air bubbles present within it. Try spraying it from a distance so as to not tamper with the bomb's composition. You must keep spraying it all through the process and not just at the last minute. Once the mixture comes together you can transfer it to the mold and keep spraying it to help it maintain form.

Shelf life

Shelf life of bath bombs will depend on the ingredients that have gone into it. But it is safe to say that most bath bombs will hold good for 6 months. You can make a tag and place it on the bottle containing the bath bomb. But don't worry, if you are making the bath bombs for children then they will get used up pretty fast and you won't have to worry about them expiring. If you drop the bomb and it emits a funny smell then it means it has passed its date.

Coloring

Some bath bombs can leave behind stains in your bathtub. This might look unsightly and deter you from using the tub. However, you can easily get rid of these stains by making use of the right ingredients. Cut a lemon wedge in half and dip it in a bowl of coarse salt. Rub this over the stain and get rid of it. You can also make use of some rubbing alcohol to rub over the stains. If nothing works then consider using strong bleach, which can assist in removing some of the stains. But use proper protection while doing so.

These form the basic mishaps that you need to know about while making bath bombs.

Chapter 9: Why You Should Make Your Own Bath Bombs

It is easy for you to buy bath bombs from stores. You will find a huge variety and buying them in bulk will work out cheap. However, there are many reasons why you should make your own bath bombs at home and some of them are as under.

Ingredients

First and foremost, you can be rest assured that the ingredients used in your bath bomb are all fresh and sourced organically. You won't have to worry about them coming from unacceptable sources. Right from the baking soda to the citric acid, you will be aware of whatever is going into the bath bombs that you are making and can confidently give it to your children to use.

Chemicals

Most commercial bath bombs can contain chemicals that

might have adverse reactions on your skin. You have to be wary of such chemicals and be a little careful while letting your children use them. Instead, you can make the bath bombs at home and eliminate any doubt. As you know, no chemicals are required to make the bath bombs and you will be able to make some with ingredients that are present within the confines of your kitchen.

Therapy

It can be viewed as a very therapeutic activity to make bath bombs. You will be able to relax, rewind and recoil while making these. You will have a fun time mixing all the ingredients, combining them well and then feeding them into molds. You will also have a great time watching them set, not to mention getting to use them. You can dedicate your weekends to making these bath bombs and put an end to your stress and tensions.

Creativity

Making bath bombs can also draw out your inner creativity. You can come up with various permutations and combinations using the different ingredients and make unique bath bombs. When your creative juices begin to flow, you will feel extremely satisfied with the end results. Don't limit yourself to the recipes mentioned in this book and keep experimenting. You will be surprised at the number of different combinations that can be achieved using the same set of oils. You can make them in small batches first to test them out and then go for the bigger batches.

Children

Getting children involved with it will help both of you have a gala time. You can get them to help you with the measurements, the mixing, and the molding process etc. you can allow them to be as creative as they like. Your children will love the activity and look forward to it. If you get good at it then you can consider hosting a workshop for their friends or children in the neighborhood. You can teach them the basics as also advanced techniques where they can learn to make bath bombs using different additives.

Gifting

It is a great idea for you to gift these bombs to others. You need not worry about finding the right gift for someone when you always have the option of giving away bath bombs. You can make a big batch, pack it neatly and give it away as a gift. You can customize it based on what the receiver likes. Some might prefer a particular color while someone else might like a particular scent. You can customize it to their liking and make the receiver extremely happy.

Cheap

As you know, bath bombs these days can cost a bomb! A single piece can set you back quite a bit and buying in bulk will mean having to spend hundreds of dollars. However, by choosing to make it at home, you can have cost effective batches. You can save on hundreds of dollars a year and remain with many different varieties of bath bombs. You just have to find the inspiration for it and start making them. You can make a list of ingredients to buy and buy them in bulk at a supermarket that allows you great discounts. Set yourself a monthly budget and use the same to remain within your spending capacity.

Environment

By choosing to make the bath bombs at home, you will be doing your bit for the environment. You won't be buying from factories that likely pollute the atmosphere. Even if there are no gases being released into the air, you will help reduce the consumption of chemicals that can harm both you and the environment. If you choose not to make use of any cling film then you will be reducing your carbon footprint as well.

Supply

When you make big batches at home, you don't have to worry about your bath bombs running out of stock. This is especially pertinent if your children don't like taking a bath without a bomb. You don't have to worry about running to the store at the last minute to buy yourself some. You can simply reach into the drawer and find a bath bomb. You can make different varieties and use a different one every day. You will never get bored of it and have an amazing time using these bath bombs while showering.

Commercial

You can consider going commercial with your hobby if you

get very good at it. If you think you know to make great bath bombs then you can consider selling them commercially. You have to etch out a plan though and know how to go about it. Start by setting yourself a budget and then come up with a menu. Advertise yourself as much as possible to get word of your business out there. Then decide upon the pricing of each unit and then give away a few samples for people to know what is on offer. Then put them up for sale and your business will be on a roll.

Remember that none of this will be possible if you buy the bombs from stores and so, it is best that you make these bath bombs by yourself.

Chapter 10: Bath Bomb Precautions

Here are some important bath bomb instructions that you have to observe in order to avoid any untoward incidents.

Smells

Some of the oils used in making bath bombs can be a bit too strong and can negatively impact those that have a sensitive predisposition to strong odors. You have to make use of those oils that aren't too strong to your family members' liking. If they are allergic to something then don't use it. Settle for something mild such as vanilla or cedar and avoid strong ones such as eucalyptus and citrus. Try dabbing some of the oil on a cotton swab and swirling it near to their noses to see how they react to it. If they sneeze or feel discomfort then don't use it.

Skin reactions

You have to be a little careful with the chemicals, as they can be a bit harsh on your skin. You have to see if they are safe for skin and only then use them. You can consider dabbing a little onto your skin and also apply some on your family members' skin. Wait for some time to see if everything is fine before going ahead with the process. If some adverse reaction takes place then wash immediately and apply a soothing cream.

Children/ elders

You have to be a little careful while using the bombs with your children. Their skin will be quite sensitive and you have to be a little careful while exposing them to things that are laden with chemicals. The same extends to elders. Their skin can be just as sensitive and you have to be careful with whatever you give them to use. Prepare a bath and test if your child's skin can handle the bath bomb before giving them a full-fledged bath. The same goes for elders in your family.

Pregnant women

It might be important for pregnant or lactating women to consult their doctors first before making use of bath bombs. They will be able to advice you on whether or not it will be safe to use them. They can contain chemicals that will penetrate your skin and you should be a little careful about it. Ask for any safer alternative soap that can help you keep your body safe.

Testing it

Stand as far back as possible when you test the bath bomb. If you are standing too close to it then you might stain your clothes. Some chemicals literally explode when they come into contact with each other or with water. You must also make sure that your children or pets are not in the same room when you test out the bath bomb. Keep a few towels and wipes ready to wipe and clean the floor if a mess ensues. It can leave the floor quite slippery which can be a bit dangerous.

Here are some things to use while making bath bombs.

Gloves

Remember to always wear gloves while making these bombs. Even if you are not using any lye or such chemicals, it is best to protect your hands. The colors and essences that you will use can be quite strong and you must protect your hands from them at all costs. Wear thick rubber gloves as compared to any plastic ones as they can adversely react to the chemicals. Remember to wash your gloves after every use in order to ready them for the next use.

Goggles

You must wear appropriate safety goggles as well to protect your eyes from some of the chemicals. These goggles can be bought at a safety equipment store and worn while both making and testing the bath bombs. They should be made from a material that is safe to be used with the chemicals and will not react adversely with them.

Apparatus

You have to buy yourself proper bath bomb making

apparatus. These will be made from materials that will not adversely react with the chemicals used in making the bath bombs. Certain plastics can cause a reaction with the chemicals and make it smell bad, which can be avoided using proper equipment. Don't use anything from the kitchen as it might make its way back there. If you are using a bowl or spoon then you must discard it immediately.

Appropriate clothing

Try wearing old clothes that you don't use anymore. You can also buy aprons that will serve the purpose. The clothes that you use should be easily washable and reusable. Wearing white is always recommended as you can easily spot any stains and get rid of them. Wearing loose clothes is also an important precaution to take as also wearing something with long sleeves.

Ventilation

There should be proper and sufficient ventilation in the room. You have to allow the chemical laden air to escape the room and also fresh air to blow in. carry out the processes in a room that contains an exhaust fan.

These form the various safety precautions to observe while choosing to make bath bombs at home.

Chapter 11: Bath Bomb Recipes

Now that you have gone over the multiple benefits of bath bombs, I am pretty sure that you are excited to make your own bath bombs! This chapter is packed with exciting bath bomb recipes, which will definitely motivate you to try them out almost at once.

Chocolate Peppermint bath bombs

Ingredients:

- 2 cups of Epsom salt
- 4 cups of baking soda
- 3 cups of cornstarch
- 1 cup of buttermilk powder
- 2 cups of citric acid
- 4 ounces of cocoa butter
- 4 ounces of vegetable glycerin
- 1 cup of honey powder
- 12 tablespoons of cocoa powder
- 4 teaspoons of peppermint essential oil

- 4 ounces of fractionated coconut oil
- 12 tablespoons of parsley powder

Instructions:

1. Take a double broiler first. Take the cocoa butter and add it to the broiler. Allow it to melt slowly.
2. Wait till the butter melts completely. Add the fractionated coconut oil and the vegetable glycerin to the broiler at this point. Mix well to ensure that the oil, glycerin and melted butter blend well. Remove the mixture from the broiler and keep it aside.
3. As the butter mixture is resting, take a large bowl. Add the Epsom salt and baking soda to it. Incorporate well with the help of your hands. Make sure that there are no lumps in the mixture.
4. Now, take the peppermint essential oil and pour it into the bowl. Mix well to ensure that the oil blends well with the baking soda mixture.
5. Next, take the citric acid, buttermilk powder, honey powder and cornstarch and add it to the bowl. Mix all the ingredients well. Once the ingredients have blended well, divide the mixture between two bowls.
6. Add the cocoa powder to one of the bowls and mix well.
7. Add the parsley powder to the other bowl and mix well.
8. Pour half the butter mixture into one of the bowls first. Knead the mixture well. Once all the ingredients have mixed well, scoop some mixture out of the bowl. Mold it in the shape of a bomb now. Repeat this step till the remaining mixture is molded in the shape of bombs.

9. Now, add the butter mixture to the other bowl. Repeat step 8 and ensure that the remainder of the mixture is shaped in the form of bombs as well.
10. Now, arrange the bombs neatly on a baking sheet. Allow them to rest for at least 24 hours. This should be sufficient time for the bombs to harden. Once they have dried completely, transfer them to airtight containers.
11. Pop a couple of bombs into your bathtub filled with warm water and enjoy a refreshing bath!

Heart bath bombs

Ingredients:

- Heart molds
- 4 cups of baking soda
- 1 cup of extra fine Epsom salt
- 2 cups of citric acid
- 2 tablespoons of jojoba oil
- 4 tablespoons of pink Brazilian clay
- Witch Hazel spray
- 12 tablespoons of grapefruit essential oil

Instructions:

1. Take a large bowl. Add the baking soda, citric acid and Epsom salt to it. Ensure that they are mixed well. This will definitely result in the formation of lumps. An easier way to get rid of these lumps would be to strain the mixture through a strainer.
2. Once the baking soda mixture is free of lumps, pour the grapefruit essential oil into the bowl next. Mix well.
3. Add the jojoba oil to the mixture in the bowl next and mix well. Keep mixing till the consistency of this mixture is that of a fine powder.
4. Divide the powdery mixture between two bowls.
5. Allow the mixture in one bowl to stay colorless.
6. Add the pink Brazilian clay to the mixture in the second bowl and mix well. Ensure that the ingredients combine well.

7. Now, take the witch hazel and spray it over the mixture in both the bowls. Knead the mixture in both the bowls well. If the mixture begins to stick together, add some jojoba oil to it and knead again.

8. Transfer the mixture to the heart shaped molds. Allow them to rest for at least 24 hours. This should be sufficient time for the bombs to harden. Once they have dried completely, transfer them to airtight containers.

9. Pop a couple of bombs into your bathtub filled with warm water and enjoy a refreshing bath!

Eucalyptus bath bombs

Ingredients:

- 1 cup of fine grind Epsom salts
- 1 cup of cornstarch
- 2 cups of baking soda
- ½ cup of cream of tartar
- 30 drops of lime essential oil
- 2 teaspoons of water
- 5 teaspoons of pure grapeseed oil
- 10 drops of green food coloring
- Silicone molds
- 20 teaspoons of eucalyptus essential oil

Instructions:

1. Take a large bowl. Add the baking soda, cornstarch, cream of tartar and Epsom salt to it. Ensure that they are mixed well.
2. Take a mixing bowl. Pour the grapeseed oil into the bowl first.
3. Add the food coloring, water, and eucalyptus essential oil and lime essential oil to the mixing bowl next and mix well. Ensure that the oils blend well.
4. Now, pour the oil mixture into the large bowl containing the baking soda mixture in a slow fashion. Use a mixer to blend all the ingredients in an even fashion.
5. Ensure that the mixture is free of lumps. Transfer the fine mixture to the silicone molds. With the help of your fingers, press the mixture into the molds firmly.

Make sure that you pack the ingredients tightly. This is important because the tighter you pack the mixture, the easier it will be to take it out of the molds.

6. Allow them to rest for at least 24 hours. This should be sufficient time for the bombs to harden. Once they have dried completely, transfer them to airtight containers.

7. Pop a couple of bombs into your bathtub filled with warm water and enjoy a refreshing bath!

Lemon bath bomb

Ingredients:

- 4 cups of cornstarch
- 4 cups of baking soda
- 4 cups of citric acid
- 1 cup of Epsom salt
- 40 drops of lemon essential oil
- Water
- 60 drops of Yellow food coloring
- Bath bomb molds

Instructions:

1. Take a large bowl. Add the baking soda, cornstarch, citric acid and Epsom salt to it. Ensure that they are mixed well.
2. Pour the lemon essential oil into the bowl next and mix well.
3. Add the yellow food coloring to the mixture and mix well.
4. Take some water and spray it over the mixture. The water will help in binding the ingredients well. Ensure that the mixture is wet enough to be pressed firmly into the molds.
5. Ensure that the mixture is free of lumps. Transfer the fine mixture to the molds. With the help of your fingers, press the mixture into the molds firmly. Make sure that you pack the ingredients tightly. This is important because the tighter you pack the mixture, the easier it will be to take it out of the molds.

6. Allow them to rest for at least 24 hours. This should be sufficient time for the bombs to harden. Once they have dried completely, transfer them to airtight containers.

7. Pop a couple of bombs into your bathtub filled with warm water and enjoy a refreshing bath!

Orange bath bombs

Ingredients:

- 2 cups of cornstarch
- 4 cups of baking soda
- 2 cups of citric acid
- 1 cup of Epsom salt
- 2 teaspoons of orange essential oil
- 4 tablespoons of water
- Orange food coloring
- Bath bomb molds

Instructions:

1. Take a large bowl. Add the baking soda, cornstarch, citric acid and Epsom salt to it. Ensure that they are mixed well.
2. Pour the orange essential oil into the bowl next and mix well.
3. Add the orange food coloring to the mixture and mix well.
4. Take some water and spray it over the mixture. The water will help in binding the ingredients well. Ensure that the mixture is wet enough to be pressed firmly into the molds.
5. Ensure that the mixture is free of lumps. Transfer the fine mixture to the molds. With the help of your fingers, press the mixture into the molds firmly. Make sure that you pack the ingredients tightly. This is important because the tighter you pack the mixture, the easier it will be to take it out of the molds.

6. Allow them to rest for at least 24 hours. This should be sufficient time for the bombs to harden. Once they have dried completely, transfer them to airtight containers.

7. Pop a couple of bombs into your bathtub filled with warm water and enjoy a refreshing bath!

Lavender bath bombs

Ingredients:

- 32 ounces of baking soda
- 16 ounces of Epsom salt
- 16 ounces of cornstarch
- 120 drops of lavender essential oil
- 16 ounces of cream of tartar
- 3 teaspoons of filtered water
- 8 teaspoons of coconut oil
- Purple or violet food coloring

Instructions:

1. Take a large bowl. Add the baking soda, cornstarch, cream of tartar and Epsom salt to it. Ensure that they are mixed well.
2. Take a mixing bowl. Pour the coconut oil into the bowl first.
3. Add the food coloring, filtered water and lavender essential oil to the mixing bowl next and mix well. Ensure that the oils blend well.
4. Now, pour the oil mixture into the large bowl containing the baking soda mixture in a slow fashion. Use a mixer to blend all the ingredients in an even fashion.
5. Ensure that the mixture is free of lumps. Transfer the fine mixture to the silicone molds. With the help of your fingers, press the mixture into the molds firmly. Make sure that you pack the ingredients tightly. This

is important because the tighter you pack the mixture, the easier it will be to take it out of the molds.

6. Allow them to rest for at least 24 hours. This should be sufficient time for the bombs to harden. Once they have dried completely, transfer them to airtight containers.

7. Pop a couple of bombs into your bathtub filled with warm water and enjoy a refreshing bath!

Eucalyptus and peppermint oil bath bomb

Ingredients:

- 20 drops of peppermint essential oil
- 4 cups of baking soda
- 20 drops of eucalyptus essential oil
- 2 cups of citric acid
- 1 cup of water
- 2 cups of cornstarch
- 1 cup of Epsom salt

Instructions:

1. Take a large bowl. Add the baking soda, cornstarch, citric acid and Epsom salt to it. Ensure that they are mixed well.
2. Take a mixing bowl. Pour the eucalyptus essential oil into the bowl first.
3. Add the water and peppermint essential oil to the mixing bowl next and mix well. Ensure that the oils blend well.
4. Now, pour the oil mixture into the large bowl containing the baking soda mixture in a slow fashion. Use a mixer to blend all the ingredients in an even fashion.
5. Ensure that the mixture is free of lumps. Transfer the fine mixture to the silicone molds. With the help of your fingers, press the mixture into the molds firmly. Make sure that you pack the ingredients tightly. This is important because the tighter you pack the mixture, the easier it will be to take it out of the molds.

6. Allow them to rest for at least 24 hours. This should be sufficient time for the bombs to harden. Once they have dried completely, transfer them to airtight containers.
7. Pop a couple of bombs into your bathtub filled with warm water and enjoy a refreshing bath! These bath bombs are also capable of clearing your sinus and relieving you from headaches.

Lavender and bergamot bath bomb

Ingredients:

- 20 drops of lavender essential oil
- 4 cups of baking soda
- 20 drops of bergamot essential oil
- 2 cups of citric acid
- 1 cup of water
- 2 cups of cornstarch
- 1 cup of Epsom salt

Instructions:

1. Take a large bowl. Add the baking soda, cornstarch, citric acid and Epsom salt to it. Ensure that they are mixed well.
2. Take a mixing bowl. Pour the lavender essential oil into the bowl first.
3. Add the water and bergamot essential oil to the mixing bowl next and mix well. Ensure that the oils blend well.
4. Now, pour the oil mixture into the large bowl containing the baking soda mixture in a slow fashion. Use a mixer to blend all the ingredients in an even fashion.
5. Ensure that the mixture is free of lumps. Transfer the fine mixture to the silicone molds. With the help of your fingers, press the mixture into the molds firmly. Make sure that you pack the ingredients tightly. This is important because the tighter you pack the mixture, the easier it will be to take it out of the molds.

6. Allow them to rest for at least 24 hours. This should be sufficient time for the bombs to harden. Once they have dried completely, transfer them to airtight containers.

7. Pop a couple of bombs into your bathtub filled with warm water and enjoy a refreshing bath! These bath bombs are capable of relaxing you and relieving you of stress.

Lemon and rosemary bath bomb

Ingredients:

- 20 drops of lemon essential oil
- 4 cups of baking soda
- 20 drops of rosemary essential oil
- 2 cups of citric acid
- 1 cup of water
- 2 cups of cornstarch
- 1 cup of Epsom salt

Instructions:

1. Take a large bowl. Add the baking soda, cornstarch, citric acid and Epsom salt to it. Ensure that they are mixed well.
2. Take a mixing bowl. Pour the lemon essential oil into the bowl first.
3. Add the water and rosemary essential oil to the mixing bowl next and mix well. Ensure that the oils blend well.
4. Now, pour the oil mixture into the large bowl containing the baking soda mixture in a slow fashion. Use a mixer to blend all the ingredients in an even fashion.
5. Ensure that the mixture is free of lumps. Transfer the fine mixture to the silicone molds. With the help of your fingers, press the mixture into the molds firmly. Make sure that you pack the ingredients tightly. This is important because the tighter you pack the mixture, the easier it will be to take it out of the molds.

6. Allow them to rest for at least 24 hours. This should be sufficient time for the bombs to harden. Once they have dried completely, transfer them to airtight containers.

7. Pop a couple of bombs into your bathtub filled with warm water and enjoy a refreshing bath! These bath bombs are capable of relaxing you and relieving you of stress.

Sage, mint and tea tree oil bath bombs

Ingredients:

- 20 drops of sage essential oil
- 4 cups of baking soda
- 10 drops of tea tree essential oil
- 1 cup of water
- 10 drops of mint essential oil
- 2 cups of citric acid
- 2 cups of cornstarch
- 1 cup of Epsom salt

Instructions:

1. Take a large bowl. Add the baking soda, cornstarch, citric acid and Epsom salt to it. Ensure that they are mixed well.
2. Take a mixing bowl. Pour the sage essential oil and tea tree essential oil into the bowl first. Ensure that the oils blend well.
3. Add the water and mint essential oil to the mixing bowl next and mix well. Ensure that the oils blend well.
4. Now, pour the oil mixture into the large bowl containing the baking soda mixture in a slow fashion. Use a mixer to blend all the ingredients in an even fashion.
5. Ensure that the mixture is free of lumps. Transfer the fine mixture to the silicone molds. With the help of your fingers, press the mixture into the molds firmly. Make sure that you pack the ingredients tightly. This

is important because the tighter you pack the mixture, the easier it will be to take it out of the molds.

6. Allow them to rest for at least 24 hours. This should be sufficient time for the bombs to harden. Once they have dried completely, transfer them to airtight containers.

7. Pop a couple of bombs into your bathtub filled with warm water and enjoy a refreshing bath! These bath bombs are capable of relaxing you and relieving you of stress.

Lavender, geranium and rose oil bath bombs

Ingredients:

- 20 drops of lavender essential oil
- 1 cup of water
- 1 cup of Epsom salt
- 10 drops of geranium essential oil
- 4 cups of baking soda
- 2 cups of citric acid
- 10 drops of rose essential oil
- 2 cups of cornstarch

Instructions:

1. Take a large bowl. Add the baking soda, cornstarch, citric acid and Epsom salt to it. Ensure that they are mixed well.
2. Take a mixing bowl. Pour the lavender essential oil and geranium essential oil into the bowl first. Mix well.
3. Add the water and rose essential oil to the mixing bowl next and mix well. Ensure that the oils blend well.
4. Now, pour the oil mixture into the large bowl containing the baking soda mixture in a slow fashion. Use a mixer to blend all the ingredients in an even fashion.
5. Ensure that the mixture is free of lumps. Transfer the fine mixture to the silicone molds. With the help of your fingers, press the mixture into the molds firmly. Make sure that you pack the ingredients tightly. This

is important because the tighter you pack the mixture, the easier it will be to take it out of the molds.

6. Allow them to rest for at least 24 hours. This should be sufficient time for the bombs to harden. Once they have dried completely, transfer them to airtight containers.

7. Pop a couple of bombs into your bathtub filled with warm water and enjoy a refreshing bath!

Cedarwood, lemon, clove and orange essential oil bath bomb

Ingredients:

- 5 drops of cedarwood essential oil
- ½ cup of Epsom salt
- 2 cups of baking soda
- 5 drops of clove essential oil
- 1 cup of citric acid
- 5 drops of lemon essential oil
- ½ cup of water
- 5 drops of orange essential oil
- 1 cup of cornstarch

Instructions:

1. Take a large bowl. Add the baking soda, cornstarch, citric acid and Epsom salt to it. Ensure that they are mixed well.
2. Take a mixing bowl. Pour the cedarwood essential oil and clove essential oil into the bowl first. Mix well.
3. Pour the lemon essential oil into the bowl next and mix well.
4. Add the water and orange essential oil to the mixing bowl next and mix well. Ensure that the oils blend well.
5. Now, pour the oil mixture into the large bowl containing the baking soda mixture in a slow fashion. Use a mixer to blend all the ingredients in an even fashion.

6. Ensure that the mixture is free of lumps. Transfer the fine mixture to the silicone molds. With the help of your fingers, press the mixture into the molds firmly. Make sure that you pack the ingredients tightly. This is important because the tighter you pack the mixture, the easier it will be to take it out of the molds.
7. Allow them to rest for at least 24 hours. This should be sufficient time for the bombs to harden. Once they have dried completely, transfer them to airtight containers.
8. Pop a couple of bombs into your bathtub filled with warm water and enjoy a refreshing bath!

Sage and lavender surprise

Ingredients:

- 64 ounces of baking soda
- 32 ounces of citric acid
- 1.2 ounces of Bentonite clay
- 40 drops of sage essential oil
- 40 drops of lavender essential oil
- 160 drops of green soap colorant
- 10 drops of olive oil
- 0.8 ounce of lavender flower powder
- 10 drops of castor oil
- Witch hazel spray

Instructions:

1. Take a large bowl. Add the baking soda, bentonite clay, citric acid and lavender flower powder to it. Ensure that they are mixed well.
2. Take a mixing bowl. Pour the sage essential oil and lavender essential oil into the bowl first. Mix well.
3. Pour the green soap colorant into the bowl next and mix well.
4. Add the castor oil and olive oil to the mixing bowl next and mix well. Ensure that the oils blend well.
5. Now, pour the oil mixture into the large bowl containing the baking soda mixture in a slow fashion. Use a mixer to blend all the ingredients in an even fashion.
6. Spray the Witch hazel over the mixture to ensure that the ingredients blend well.

7. Ensure that the mixture is free of lumps. Transfer the fine mixture to the silicone molds. With the help of your fingers, press the mixture into the molds firmly. Make sure that you pack the ingredients tightly. This is important because the tighter you pack the mixture, the easier it will be to take it out of the molds.
8. Allow them to rest for at least 24 hours. This should be sufficient time for the bombs to harden. Once they have dried completely, transfer them to airtight containers.
9. Pop a couple of bombs into your bathtub filled with warm water and enjoy a refreshing bath!

Gold, myrrh and frankincense bath bombs

Ingredients:

- 2 cups of baking soda
- 1 1/3 cups of Epsom salt
- 1 teaspoon of gold mica
- 80 drops of frankincense essential oil
- Water
- 20 drops of myrrh essential oil
- 2 tablespoons of Turkey red oil
- 1 cup of citric acid

Instructions:

1. Take a food processor. Add the mica, baking soda and Epsom salts to the bowl of the processor first.
2. Pour the Turkey red oil, myrrh essential oil and frankincense essential oil into the bowl next. Blend the ingredients well and transfer the mixture to a large bowl.
3. Now, add the citric acid to the bowl and mix well.
4. Now, take some water and spray it over the mixture. The water will help in binding the ingredients well. Ensure that the mixture is wet enough to be pressed firmly into the molds.
5. Ensure that the mixture is free of lumps. Transfer the fine mixture to the molds. With the help of your fingers, press the mixture into the molds firmly. Make sure that you pack the ingredients tightly. This is important because the tighter you pack the mixture, the easier it will be to take it out of the molds.

6. Allow them to rest for at least 24 hours. This should be sufficient time for the bombs to harden. Once they have dried completely, transfer them to airtight containers.
7. Pop a couple of bombs into your bathtub filled with warm water and enjoy a refreshing bath!

Green tea bath bomb

Ingredients:

- 4 cups of baking soda
- 2 cups of citric acid
- 8 tablespoons of Matcha (powdered green tea)
- 1 teaspoon of lavender essential oil
- 1 cup of Epsom salt
- 8 tablespoons of almond oil
- 1 cup of cornstarch
- 8 teaspoons of water

Instructions:

1. Take a large bowl. Add the baking soda, cornstarch, citric acid and Epsom salt to it. Ensure that they are mixed well.
2. Add the Matcha to the baking soda mixture and mix well.
3. Pour the almond oil and lavender essential oil into the bowl next. Mix well to ensure that the ingredients blend well.
4. Now, take some water and spray it over the mixture. The water will help in binding the ingredients well. Ensure that the mixture is wet enough to be pressed firmly into the molds.
5. Ensure that the mixture is free of lumps. Transfer the fine mixture to the molds. With the help of your fingers, press the mixture into the molds firmly. Make sure that you pack the ingredients tightly. This is

important because the tighter you pack the mixture, the easier it will be to take it out of the molds.

6. Allow them to rest for at least 24 hours. This should be sufficient time for the bombs to harden. Once they have dried completely, transfer them to airtight containers.

7. Pop a couple of bombs into your bathtub filled with warm water and enjoy a refreshing bath!

Grapefruit bath bomb

Ingredients:

- 4 cups of baking soda
- 4 teaspoons of water
- 12 tablespoons of coconut oil
- 2 cups of citric acid
- 4 teaspoons of beet juice
- 16 drops of grapefruit essential oil
- 8 tablespoons of Epsom salt

Instructions:

1. Take a double broiler first. Take the coconut oil and add it to the broiler. Allow it to melt slowly.
2. Wait till the oil melts completely. Upon the oil melting, remove it from the broiler and keep it aside.
3. As the oil is resting, take a large bowl. Add the baking soda, citric acid and Epsom salt to it. Ensure that they are mixed well.
4. Take a mixing bowl. Pour the coconut oil and grapefruit essential oil into the bowl first. Mix well.
5. Add the beet juice to the mixing bowl next and mix well. Ensure that the juice and the oils blend well.
6. Now, pour the oil mixture into the large bowl containing the baking soda mixture in a slow fashion. Use a mixer to blend all the ingredients in an even fashion.
7. Now, take water and spray it over the mixture. The water will help in binding the ingredients well. Ensure that the mixture is wet enough to be pressed firmly into the molds.

8. Ensure that the mixture is free of lumps. Transfer the fine mixture to the silicone molds. With the help of your fingers, press the mixture into the molds firmly. Make sure that you pack the ingredients tightly. This is important because the tighter you pack the mixture, the easier it will be to take it out of the molds.
9. Allow them to rest for at least 24 hours. This should be sufficient time for the bombs to harden. Once they have dried completely, transfer them to airtight containers.
10. Pop a couple of bombs into your bathtub filled with warm water and enjoy a refreshing bath!

Honey and milk heart treats

Ingredients:

- 8 cups of baking soda
- 12 tablespoons of honey powder
- 4 cups of citric acid
- 12 tablespoons of whole milk powder
- 12 tablespoons of oatmeal
- 8 ounces of Witch Hazel
- 12 tablespoons of chamomile flower powder
- 4 teaspoons of frankincense essential oil

Instructions:

1. Take a large bowl. Add the baking soda and frankincense essential oil to it. Ensure that they are mixed well.
2. Now, add the honey powder and chamomile flower powder to the bowl and mix well.
3. Next, add the oatmeal and whole milk powder to the bowl and mix well.
4. Add the citric acid to the bowl next and mix well.
5. Now, take the Witch Hazel and spray it over the mixture. The spray will help in binding the ingredients well. Ensure that the mixture is wet enough to be pressed firmly into the molds.
6. Ensure that the mixture is free of lumps. Transfer the fine mixture to the molds. With the help of your fingers, press the mixture into the molds firmly. Make sure that you pack the ingredients tightly. This is

important because the tighter you pack the mixture, the easier it will be to take it out of the molds.

7. Allow them to rest for at least 24 hours. This should be sufficient time for the bombs to harden. Once they have dried completely, transfer them to airtight containers.

8. Pop a couple of bombs into your bathtub filled with warm water and enjoy a refreshing bath!

Aloe bubble bath bomb

Ingredients:

- 20 ounces of aloe extract
- 2 cups of sodium Lauryl Sulfoacetate
- 4 cups of baking soda
- 8 leaf wax tart molds
- ½ ounce Kentish rain fragrance oil
- Irish green colorant
- Witch Hazel
- ¼ ounce of Basmati rice fragrance oil
- 2 cups of citric acid

Instructions:

1. Take a large bowl. Add the baking soda and citric acid to it. Ensure that they are mixed well.
2. Now, add the sodium lauryl sulfoacetate to the baking soda mixture. Using your hands, ensure that the sulfoacetate mixes well with the mixture. Care should be exercised while carrying out this step since the sodium lauryl sulfoacetate can be quite powerful. Hence, ensure that you are in a nicely ventilated room, when you carry out this. To avoid sneezing, you may also opt for wearing a surgical mask.
3. Take the colorant next and add it to the mixture in the bowl, one drop at a time. Continue to add the drops till the color of the baking soda mixture is minty green. Do remember that more the number of drops you add, the more colorful your bath will be. Hence,

do not add too much if you don't want your water to be too colorful.

4. Now that the color of the mixture has changed to green, take the aloe extract and add it to the bowl.

5. Pour the rain fragrance oil into the bowl next and mix well.

6. Take the Basmati rice fragrance oil and add it to the bowl next. Mix well.

7. If you find that the consistency of your mixture is a bit dry and powdery, spray some Witch hazel over it. This will ensure that the ingredients bind well. In order to ensure that the ingredients bind well, you may have to spray it at least ten times over the mixture.

8. Ensure that the mixture is free of lumps. Transfer the fine mixture to the wax tart molds. With the help of your fingers, press the mixture into the molds firmly. Make sure that you pack the ingredients tightly. This is important because the tighter you pack the mixture, the easier it will be to take it out of the molds.

9. Allow them to rest for at least 24 hours. This should be sufficient time for the bombs to harden. Once they have dried completely, transfer them to airtight containers.

10. Pop a couple of bombs into your bathtub filled with warm water and enjoy a refreshing bath!

Oatmeal bath bomb

Ingredients:

- 2 ½ cups of baking soda
- 30 drops of lemon essential oil
- 1 cup of citric acid
- 4 tablespoons of water
- ½ cup of oatmeal
- 10 drops of food coloring
- 4 to 12 teaspoons of almond oil

Instructions:

1. Take a large bowl. Add the baking soda, oatmeal and citric acid to it. Ensure that they are mixed well.
2. Add the food coloring to the baking soda mixture and mix well.
3. Take a mixing bowl. Pour the lemon essential oil and almond oil into the bowl first. Mix well. Ensure that the oils blend well.
4. Now, pour the oil mixture into the large bowl containing the baking soda mixture in a slow fashion. Use a mixer to blend all the ingredients in an even fashion.
5. Now, take some water and spray it over the mixture. The water will help in binding the ingredients well. Ensure that the mixture is wet enough to be pressed firmly into the molds.
6. Ensure that the mixture is free of lumps. Transfer the fine mixture to the silicone molds. With the help of your fingers, press the mixture into the molds firmly. Make sure that you pack the ingredients tightly. This

is important because the tighter you pack the mixture, the easier it will be to take it out of the molds.

7. Allow them to rest for at least 24 hours. This should be sufficient time for the bombs to harden. Once they have dried completely, transfer them to airtight containers.

8. Pop a couple of bombs into your bathtub filled with warm water and enjoy a refreshing bath!

Blueberry bath bomb recipe

Ingredients:

- 2.4 ounces of sweet almond oil
- 154 ounces of baking soda
- 64 ounces of citric acid
- 160 drops of blueberry fragrance oil
- 1.2 ounces of ultramarine blue colorant
- 0.8 ounce of fruit powder
- Witch Hazel

Instructions:

1. Take a large bowl. Add the baking soda and citric acid to it. Ensure that they are mixed well.
2. Add the fruit powder to the baking soda mixture and mix well.
3. Take the colorant next and add it to the mixture in the bowl, one drop at a time. Continue to add the drops till the color of the baking soda mixture is blue. Do remember that more the number of drops you add, the more colorful your bath will be. Hence, do not add too much if you don't want your water to be too colorful.
4. Now that the color of the mixture has changed to blue, take the aloe extract and add it to the bowl.
5. Take a mixing bowl. Pour the blueberry fragrance oil and sweet almond oil into the bowl first. Mix well. Ensure that the oils blend well.
6. Now, pour the oil mixture into the large bowl containing the baking soda mixture in a slow fashion.

Use a mixer to blend all the ingredients in an even fashion.

7. Now, take some witch hazel and spray it over the mixture. The water will help in binding the ingredients well. Ensure that the mixture is wet enough to be pressed firmly into the molds.

8. Ensure that the mixture is free of lumps. Transfer the fine mixture to the silicone molds. With the help of your fingers, press the mixture into the molds firmly. Make sure that you pack the ingredients tightly. This is important because the tighter you pack the mixture, the easier it will be to take it out of the molds.

9. Allow them to rest for at least 24 hours. This should be sufficient time for the bombs to harden. Once they have dried completely, transfer them to airtight containers.

10. Pop a couple of bombs into your bathtub filled with warm water and enjoy a refreshing bath!

Apricot bath bombs

Ingredients:

- 4 cups of cornstarch
- 1 cup of Epsom salt
- Orange food coloring
- 4 cups of baking soda
- 2 cups of Apricot fragrance oil
- 4 cups of citric acid
- Water

Instructions:

1. Take a large bowl. Add the baking soda, cornstarch, Epsom salt and citric acid to it. Ensure that they are mixed well.
2. Add the orange food coloring to the baking soda mixture and mix well.
3. Add the apricot fragrance oil to the mixture next and mix well. Use a mixer to blend all the ingredients in an even fashion.
4. Now, take some water and spray it over the mixture. The water will help in binding the ingredients well. Ensure that the mixture is wet enough to be pressed firmly into the molds.
5. Ensure that the mixture is free of lumps. Transfer the fine mixture to the silicone molds. With the help of your fingers, press the mixture into the molds firmly. Make sure that you pack the ingredients tightly. This is important because the tighter you pack the mixture, the easier it will be to take it out of the molds.

6. Allow them to rest for at least 24 hours. This should be sufficient time for the bombs to harden. Once they have dried completely, transfer them to airtight containers.

7. Pop a couple of bombs into your bathtub filled with warm water and enjoy a refreshing bath!

White tree coconut oil bath bomb

Ingredients:

- 2 cups of cornstarch
- 8 tablespoons of coconut oil
- 2 cups of citric acid
- 4 cups of baking soda
- 24 teaspoons of white tea
- 8 tablespoons of Epsom salt
- Water

Instructions:

1. Take a large bowl. Add the baking soda, cornstarch, Epsom salt and citric acid to it. Ensure that they are mixed well.
2. Take a mixing bowl. Pour the coconut oil and white tea into the bowl first. Mix well. Ensure that the oils blend well.
3. Now, pour the oil mixture into the large bowl containing the baking soda mixture in a slow fashion. Use a mixer to blend all the ingredients in an even fashion.
4. Now, take some water and spray it over the mixture. The water will help in binding the ingredients well. Ensure that the mixture is wet enough to be pressed firmly into the molds.
5. Ensure that the mixture is free of lumps. Transfer the fine mixture to the silicone molds. With the help of your fingers, press the mixture into the molds firmly. Make sure that you pack the ingredients tightly. This

is important because the tighter you pack the mixture, the easier it will be to take it out of the molds.

6. Allow them to rest for at least 24 hours. This should be sufficient time for the bombs to harden. Once they have dried completely, transfer them to airtight containers.

7. Pop a couple of bombs into your bathtub filled with warm water and enjoy a refreshing bath!

Ginger peach bath bomb

Ingredients:

- 8 teaspoons of ginger peach fragrance oil
- 2 cups of cornstarch
- 4 cups of baking soda
- 2 cups of Epsom salt
- 2 cups of citric acid
- 8 drops of yellow food coloring
- 10 tablespoons of cherry kernel oil
- 4 drops of red food coloring
- Water

Instructions:

1. Take a large bowl. Add the baking soda, cornstarch, Epsom salt and citric acid to it. Ensure that they are mixed well.
2. Add the yellow food coloring to the mixture next and mix well. Ensure that it is well incorporated in the baking soda mixture.
3. Take the red food coloring next and add it to the mixture next. Ensure that it mixes well.
4. Take a mixing bowl. Pour the cherry kernel oil and ginger peach fragrance oil into the bowl. Mix well. Ensure that the oils blend well.
5. Now, pour the oil mixture into the large bowl containing the baking soda mixture in a slow fashion. Use a mixer to blend all the ingredients in an even fashion.

6. Now, take some water and spray it over the mixture. The water will help in binding the ingredients well. Ensure that the mixture is wet enough to be pressed firmly into the molds.

7. Ensure that the mixture is free of lumps. Transfer the fine mixture to the silicone molds. With the help of your fingers, press the mixture into the molds firmly. Make sure that you pack the ingredients tightly. This is important because the tighter you pack the mixture, the easier it will be to take it out of the molds.

8. Allow them to rest for at least 24 hours. This should be sufficient time for the bombs to harden. Once they have dried completely, transfer them to airtight containers.

9. Pop a couple of bombs into your bathtub filled with warm water and enjoy a refreshing bath!

Salty caramel bath bombs

Ingredients:

- 4 cups of cornstarch
- 8 cups of baking soda
- 4 cups of citric acid
- Few drops of food coloring
- 8 teaspoons of salty caramel ice cream fragrance oil
- 4 cups of Epsom salt
- 8 teaspoons of jojoba oil
- Water

Instructions:

1. Take a large bowl. Add the baking soda, cornstarch, Epsom salt and citric acid to it. Ensure that they are mixed well.
2. Add the food coloring to the mixture next and mix well. Ensure that it is well incorporated in the baking soda mixture.
3. Take a mixing bowl. Pour the jojoba oil and salty caramel ice cream fragrance oil into the bowl. Mix well. Ensure that the oils blend well.
4. Now, pour the oil mixture into the large bowl containing the baking soda mixture in a slow fashion. Use a mixer to blend all the ingredients in an even fashion.
5. Now, take some water and spray it over the mixture. The water will help in binding the ingredients well. Ensure that the mixture is wet enough to be pressed firmly into the molds.

6. Ensure that the mixture is free of lumps. Transfer the fine mixture to the silicone molds. With the help of your fingers, press the mixture into the molds firmly. Make sure that you pack the ingredients tightly. This is important because the tighter you pack the mixture, the easier it will be to take it out of the molds.
7. Allow them to rest for at least 24 hours. This should be sufficient time for the bombs to harden. Once they have dried completely, transfer them to airtight containers.
8. Pop a couple of bombs into your bathtub filled with warm water and enjoy a refreshing bath!

Rose and bergamot bath bomb

Ingredients:

- 4 cups of baking soda
- 20 drops of rose essential oil
- 20 drops of bergamot essential oil
- 1 cup of water
- 2 cups of citric acid
- 2 cups of cornstarch
- 1 cup of Epsom salt

Instructions:

1. Take a large bowl. Add the baking soda, cornstarch, Epsom salt and citric acid to it. Ensure that they are mixed well.
2. Take a mixing bowl. Pour the bergamot essential oil and rose essential oil into the bowl. Mix well. Ensure that the oils blend well.
3. Now, pour the oil mixture into the large bowl containing the baking soda mixture in a slow fashion. Use a mixer to blend all the ingredients in an even fashion.
4. Now, take some water and spray it over the mixture. The water will help in binding the ingredients well. Ensure that the mixture is wet enough to be pressed firmly into the molds.
5. Ensure that the mixture is free of lumps. Transfer the fine mixture to the silicone molds. With the help of your fingers, press the mixture into the molds firmly. Make sure that you pack the ingredients tightly. This

is important because the tighter you pack the mixture, the easier it will be to take it out of the molds.

6. Allow them to rest for at least 24 hours. This should be sufficient time for the bombs to harden. Once they have dried completely, transfer them to airtight containers.

7. Pop a couple of bombs into your bathtub filled with warm water and enjoy a refreshing bath!

Strawberry Shake bath bomb

Ingredients:

- 8 cups of baking soda
- 2 ounces of strawberry shake fragrance oil
- 4 cups of citric acid
- Witch hazel

Instructions:

1. Take a large bowl first. Add the baking soda to it.
2. Add the citric acid to the bowl next and mix well.
3. Take the strawberry shake fragrance oil next and pour it into the bowl in a slow fashion. Ensure that it mixes well with the baking soda mixture. Ensure that the mixture is free of lumps. Use your hands to get rid of lumps in the mixture.
4. If you find that the consistency of the mixture is too powdery and dry to your liking, spray some witch hazel over the mixture. This will ensure that the ingredients bind well. In order to ensure that the ingredients bind well, you may have to spray it at least ten times over the mixture.
5. Transfer the fine mixture to the molds. With the help of your fingers, press the mixture into the molds firmly. Make sure that you pack the ingredients tightly. This is important because the tighter you pack the mixture, the easier it will be to take it out of the molds.
6. Allow them to rest for at least 24 hours. This should be sufficient time for the bombs to harden. Once they

have dried completely, transfer them to airtight containers.

7. Pop a couple of bombs into your bathtub filled with warm water and enjoy a refreshing bath!

Cotton Candy bath bomb

Ingredients:

- 36 ounces of citric Acid
- 18 ounces of cornstarch
- 0.52 ounce of neon pink soap colorant
- 1.6 ounces of Bentonite Clay
- 1.6 ounces of Castor Oil
- 84 ounces of baking soda
- 160 drops of Cotton Candy Fragrance Oil
- 0.52 ounce of neon blue soap colorant
- Witch Hazel
- 0.26 ounce of Sweet Almond Oil

Instructions:

1. Take 4 medium sized bowls and arrange them in your work area. You would be requiring one for the dry ingredients, one for the wet ingredients and two for the colorings.
2. Add the cornstarch, baking soda and citric acid to one of the bowls. Mix the ingredients well. Ensure that the mixture is free of lumps. Should you find any lumps, use your hands to break them off. Allow this mixture to rest.
3. As the baking soda mixture is resting, take your second bowl. Add the castor oil, sweet almond oil and cotton candy fragrance oil to it and mix well. Ensure that the oils blend well.
4. Add around 20 ounces of the baking soda mixture to each of the remaining two empty bowls.

5. Add the neon blue soap colorant to the third bowl and mix well. Ensure that the mixture is evenly colored.

6. Now, add the neon pink soap colorant to the fourth bowl and mix well. Ensure that the mixture is evenly colored.

7. Now, add the oil mixture to the remaining baking soda mixture in the first bowl. Use a mixer to ensure that the ingredients blend well.

8. If you find that the consistency of the mixture is too powdery and dry to your liking, spray some witch hazel over the mixture. This will ensure that the ingredients bind well. In order to ensure that the ingredients bind well, you may have to spray it at least ten times over the mixture.

9. Now, slowly add the pink colored mixture and blue colored mixture to the bowl. Mix well. Ensure that the mixture is free of lumps. Should you find any lumps, use your hands to break them off.

10. Transfer the fine mixture to the molds. With the help of your fingers, press the mixture into the molds firmly. Make sure that you pack the ingredients tightly. This is important because the tighter you pack the mixture, the easier it will be to take it out of the molds.

11. Allow them to rest for at least 24 hours. This should be sufficient time for the bombs to harden. Once they have dried completely, transfer them to airtight containers.

12. Pop a couple of bombs into your bathtub filled with warm water and enjoy a refreshing bath!

Freshly ground coffee bath bombs

Ingredients:

- 4 ounces of apricot kernel oil
- 1 ounce of coffee grounds
- 18 ounces of citric acid
- 1.2 ounces of freshly brewed coffee fragrance oil
- 36 ounces of baking soda
- 0.6 ounce of Bentonite clay
- Witch Hazel

Instructions:

1. Before we get started with the preparation of the bath bombs, let us just take a couple of minutes to prepare the molds. Take some coffee grounds and add it to each of the molds. Keep aside.
2. Take a large bowl. Add the baking soda, Bentonite clay and citric acid to it. Ensure that they are mixed well.
3. Take a mixing bowl. Pour the coffee fragrance oil and apricot kernel oil into the bowl. Mix well. Ensure that the oils blend well.
4. Now, pour the oil mixture into the large bowl containing the baking soda mixture in a slow fashion. Use a mixer to blend all the ingredients in an even fashion.
5. Add the coffee grounds to the mixture next. Ensure that they mix well.
6. If you find that the consistency of the mixture is too powdery and dry to your liking, spray some witch hazel over the mixture. This will ensure that the

ingredients bind well. In order to ensure that the ingredients bind well, you may have to spray it at least ten times over the mixture.

7. Ensure that the mixture is free of lumps. Transfer the fine mixture to the silicone molds. With the help of your fingers, press the mixture into the molds firmly. Make sure that you pack the ingredients tightly. This is important because the tighter you pack the mixture, the easier it will be to take it out of the molds.

8. Allow them to rest for at least 24 hours. This should be sufficient time for the bombs to harden. Once they have dried completely, transfer them to airtight containers.

9. Pop a couple of bombs into your bathtub filled with warm water and enjoy a refreshing bath!

Black cherry bath bombs

Ingredients:

- 1.2 ounces of Bentonite Clay
- 158 ounces of baking soda
- 1.4 ounce of Olive Oil
- 72 ounces of citric acid
- 160 drops of black cherry bomb fragrance oil
- 2 ounces of Castor Oil
- 1.2 ounce of beet root powder
- Witch Hazel

Instructions:

1. Take a large bowl. Add the baking soda, Bentonite clay and citric acid to it. Ensure that they are mixed well.
2. Add the beetroot powder to the bowl next and mix well.
3. Take a mixing bowl. Pour the olive oil and castor oil into the bowl. Mix well. Ensure that the oils blend well.
4. Add the black cherry bomb fragrance oil to the oil mixture in the bowl and mix well.
5. Now, pour the oil mixture into the large bowl containing the baking soda mixture in a slow fashion. Use a mixer to blend all the ingredients in an even fashion.
6. If you find that the consistency of the mixture is too powdery and dry to your liking, spray some witch hazel over the mixture. This will ensure that the

ingredients bind well. In order to ensure that the ingredients bind well, you may have to spray it at least ten times over the mixture.

7. Ensure that the mixture is free of lumps. Transfer the fine mixture to the silicone molds. With the help of your fingers, press the mixture into the molds firmly. Make sure that you pack the ingredients tightly. This is important because the tighter you pack the mixture, the easier it will be to take it out of the molds.

8. Allow them to rest for at least 24 hours. This should be sufficient time for the bombs to harden. Once they have dried completely, transfer them to airtight containers.

9. Pop a couple of bombs into your bathtub filled with warm water and enjoy a refreshing bath!

Green apple bath bomb

Ingredients:

- 18 ounces of citric acid
- 36 ounces of baking soda
- 3.8 ounces of apricot kernel oil
- 0.8 ounce of Bentonite clay
- 2 ounces of Epsom salt
- 1 ounce of neon green soap colorant
- 1.2 ounces of green apple candy fragrance oil
- 12 drops of Kelly green soap colorant
- Witch Hazel

Instructions:

1. Take a large bowl. Add the baking soda, Bentonite clay and citric acid to it. Ensure that they are mixed well.
2. Add the neon green soap colorant to the baking soda mixture. Ensure that the coloring is well incorporated in the mixture.
3. Add the Kelly green soap colorant to the mixture and mix well.
4. Take a mixing bowl. Pour the apricot kernel oil and green apple candy fragrance oil into the bowl. Mix well. Ensure that the oils blend well.
5. Now, pour the oil mixture into the large bowl containing the baking soda mixture in a slow fashion. Use a mixer to blend all the ingredients in an even fashion.

6. If you find that the consistency of the mixture is too powdery and dry to your liking, spray some witch hazel over the mixture. This will ensure that the ingredients bind well. In order to ensure that the ingredients bind well, you may have to spray it at least ten times over the mixture.

7. Ensure that the mixture is free of lumps. Transfer the fine mixture to the silicone molds. With the help of your fingers, press the mixture into the molds firmly. Make sure that you pack the ingredients tightly. This is important because the tighter you pack the mixture, the easier it will be to take it out of the molds.

8. Allow them to rest for at least 24 hours. This should be sufficient time for the bombs to harden. Once they have dried completely, transfer them to airtight containers.

9. Pop a couple of bombs into your bathtub filled with warm water and enjoy a refreshing bath!

Orange dreamsickle bath bomb

Ingredients:

- 79 ounces of baking soda
- 36 ounces of citric acid
- 1.3 ounces of sweet almond oil
- 28 drops of eye poke orange soap colorant
- 40 drops of dreamsickle fragrance oil
- 0.4 ounce of vanilla powder
- 0.2 ounce of orange peel powder
- Witch Hazel

Instructions:

1. Take a large bowl. Add the baking soda, Bentonite clay and citric acid to it. Ensure that they are mixed well.
2. Add the orange peel powder and vanilla powder to the mixture and mix well.
3. Add the eye poke orange soap colorant to the baking soda mixture. Ensure that the coloring is well incorporated in the mixture.
4. Take a mixing bowl. Pour the sweet almond oil and dreamsickle fragrance oil into the bowl. Mix well. Ensure that the oils blend well.
5. Now, pour the oil mixture into the large bowl containing the baking soda mixture in a slow fashion. Use a mixer to blend all the ingredients in an even fashion.
6. If you find that the consistency of the mixture is too powdery and dry to your liking, spray some

witch hazel over the mixture. This will ensure that the ingredients bind well. In order to ensure that the ingredients bind well, you may have to spray it at least ten times over the mixture.

7. Ensure that the mixture is free of lumps. Transfer the fine mixture to the silicone molds. With the help of your fingers, press the mixture into the molds firmly. Make sure that you pack the ingredients tightly. This is important because the tighter you pack the mixture, the easier it will be to take it out of the molds.

8. Allow them to rest for at least 24 hours. This should be sufficient time for the bombs to harden. Once they have dried completely, transfer them to airtight containers.

9. Pop a couple of bombs into your bathtub filled with warm water and enjoy a refreshing bath!

Wild bath bomb

Ingredients:

- 18 ounces of citric acid
- 36 ounces of baking soda
- 4 ounces of coconut oil
- 0.6 ounce of orange oxide soap colorant
- 0.8 ounce of Kaolin clay
- 0.4 ounce of eye poke orange soap colorant
- Witch Hazel
- 1.2 ounces of ferocious beast fragrance oil

Instructions:

1. Take a large bowl. Add the baking soda, Kaolin clay and citric acid to it. Ensure that they are mixed well.
2. Add the orange oxide soap colorant to the baking soda mixture first. Ensure that it mixes well.
3. Add the eye poke orange soap colorant to the baking soda mixture. Ensure that the coloring is well incorporated in the mixture.
4. Take a mixing bowl. Pour the coconut oil and ferocious beast fragrance oil into the bowl. Mix well. Ensure that the oils blend well.
5. Now, pour the oil mixture into the large bowl containing the baking soda mixture in a slow fashion. Use a mixer to blend all the ingredients in an even fashion.
6. If you find that the consistency of the mixture is too powdery and dry to your liking, spray some

witch hazel over the mixture. This will ensure that the ingredients bind well. In order to ensure that the ingredients bind well, you may have to spray it at least ten times over the mixture.

7. Ensure that the mixture is free of lumps. Transfer the fine mixture to the silicone molds. With the help of your fingers, press the mixture into the molds firmly. Make sure that you pack the ingredients tightly. This is important because the tighter you pack the mixture, the easier it will be to take it out of the molds.

8. Allow them to rest for at least 24 hours. This should be sufficient time for the bombs to harden. Once they have dried completely, transfer them to airtight containers.

9. Pop a couple of bombs into your bathtub filled with warm water and enjoy a refreshing bath!

Sinus relief bath bomb

Ingredients:

- 0.6 ounce of Bentonite Clay
- 36 ounces of citric acid
- 79 ounces of baking soda
- 80 drops of sinus relief fragrance oil
- 0.9 ounce of Castor Oil
- 0.2 ounce of peppermint leaf powder
- 0.7 ounce of Olive Oil
- 0.07 ounce of chopped spearmint leaves
- Witch Hazel

Instructions:

1. Take a large bowl. Add the baking soda, Bentonite clay and citric acid to it. Ensure that they are mixed well.
2. Add the peppermint leaf powder to the mixture next and mix well.
3. Take the chopped spearmint leaves next and add it to the mixture. Ensure that the ingredients blend well.
4. Take a mixing bowl. Pour the olive oil and castor oil into the bowl. Mix well. Ensure that the oils blend well.
5. Add the sinus relief fragrance oil to the oil mixture next. Mix well.
6. Now, pour the oil mixture into the large bowl containing the baking soda mixture in a slow

fashion. Use a mixer to blend all the ingredients in an even fashion.

7. If you find that the consistency of the mixture is too powdery and dry to your liking, spray some witch hazel over the mixture. This will ensure that the ingredients bind well. In order to ensure that the ingredients bind well, you may have to spray it at least ten times over the mixture.

8. Ensure that the mixture is free of lumps. Transfer the fine mixture to the silicone molds. With the help of your fingers, press the mixture into the molds firmly. Make sure that you pack the ingredients tightly. This is important because the tighter you pack the mixture, the easier it will be to take it out of the molds.

9. Allow them to rest for at least 24 hours. This should be sufficient time for the bombs to harden. Once they have dried completely, transfer them to airtight containers.

10. Pop a couple of bombs into your bathtub filled with warm water and enjoy a refreshing bath!

Gingersnap cookies bath bombs

Ingredients:

- 8 cups of baking soda
- 4 cups of citric acid
- 2 ounces of gingersnap cookies fragrance oil
- 160 drops of brown soap coloring
- Witch Hazel

Instructions:

1. Take a large bowl. Add the baking soda clay and citric acid to it. Ensure that they are mixed well.
2. Add the gingersnap cookies fragrance oil to the bowl next. Ensure that the oil mixes well with the baking soda mixture. Ensure that there are no lumps. Should you find any, use your hand to break off these.
3. Add the brown soap coloring to the mixture next. Use a mixer to blend all the ingredients in an even fashion.
4. If you find that the consistency of the mixture is too powdery and dry to your liking, spray some witch hazel over the mixture. This will ensure that the ingredients bind well. In order to ensure that the ingredients bind well, you may have to spray it at least ten times over the mixture.
5. Ensure that the mixture is free of lumps. Transfer the fine mixture to the silicone molds. With the help of your fingers, press the mixture into the molds firmly. Make sure that you pack the ingredients tightly. This is important because the

tighter you pack the mixture, the easier it will be to take it out of the molds.

6. Allow them to rest for at least 24 hours. This should be sufficient time for the bombs to harden. Once they have dried completely, transfer them to airtight containers.

7. Pop a couple of bombs into your bathtub filled with warm water and enjoy a refreshing bath!

Pink salt bath bombs

Ingredients:

- 9 ounces of citric acid
- 2 ounces of coconut oil
- 18 ounces of baking soda
- 0.3 ounce of Bentonite clay
- 2 ounces of finely ground Himalayan pink salt
- 5 ounces of cornstarch
- 0.07 ounce of Che belladonna fragrance oil
- 2 ounces of coarsely ground Himalayan pink salt
- 0.3 ounce of neon pink soap colorant

Instructions:

1. Before we get started with the preparation of the bath bombs, let us just take a couple of minutes to prepare the molds. Sprinkle the coarsely ground Himalayan pink salt over each of the molds. Keep aside.
2. Take a large bowl. Add the baking soda, cornstarch, finely ground Himalayan pink salt, Bentonite clay and citric acid to it. Ensure that they are mixed well.
3. Take a mixing bowl. Pour the coconut oil and Che belladonna fragrance oil into the bowl. Mix well. Ensure that the oils blend well.
4. Add the neon pink soap colorant to the oil mixture and mix well.
5. Now, pour the oil mixture into the large bowl containing the baking soda mixture in a slow fashion. Use a mixer to blend all the ingredients in an even fashion.

6. If you find that the consistency of the mixture is too powdery and dry to your liking, spray some witch hazel over the mixture. This will ensure that the ingredients bind well. In order to ensure that the ingredients bind well, you may have to spray it at least ten times over the mixture.

7. Ensure that the mixture is free of lumps. Transfer the fine mixture to the silicone molds. With the help of your fingers, press the mixture into the molds firmly. Make sure that you pack the ingredients tightly. This is important because the tighter you pack the mixture, the easier it will be to take it out of the molds.

8. Allow them to rest for at least 24 hours. This should be sufficient time for the bombs to harden. Once they have dried completely, transfer them to airtight containers.

9. Pop a couple of bombs into your bathtub filled with warm water and enjoy a refreshing bath!

Jasmine bath bomb

Ingredients:

- 4 cups of baking soda
- 1 1/3 cups of Epsom salt
- 2 cups of citric acid
- 2 cups of cornstarch
- 10 tablespoons of sweet almond oil
- 4 teaspoons of vitamin E oil
- 3 tablespoons of water
- 1 teaspoon of jasmine fragrance oil
- Witch hazel
- 1 teaspoon of borax
- Food coloring

Instructions:

1. Take a large bowl. Add the baking soda, cornstarch, Epsom salts and citric acid to it. Ensure that they are mixed well.
2. Add the borax to the mixture next and mix well.
3. Take a mixing bowl. Pour the water and sweet almond oil into the bowl. Mix well. Ensure that the oils blend well.
4. Add the jasmine fragrance oil to the oil mixture next. Mix well.
5. Add the vitamin E oil to the oil mixture and mix well.
6. Take the food coloring and add it to the oil mixture next. Make sure that the food coloring blends well with the oil mixture.

7. Now, pour the oil mixture into the large bowl containing the baking soda mixture in a slow fashion. Use a mixer to blend all the ingredients in an even fashion.

8. If you find that the consistency of the mixture is too powdery and dry to your liking, spray some witch hazel over the mixture. This will ensure that the ingredients bind well. In order to ensure that the ingredients bind well, you may have to spray it at least ten times over the mixture.

9. Ensure that the mixture is free of lumps. Transfer the fine mixture to the silicone molds. With the help of your fingers, press the mixture into the molds firmly. Make sure that you pack the ingredients tightly. This is important because the tighter you pack the mixture, the easier it will be to take it out of the molds.

10. Allow them to rest for at least 24 hours. This should be sufficient time for the bombs to harden. Once they have dried completely, transfer them to airtight containers.

11. Pop a couple of bombs into your bathtub filled with warm water and enjoy a refreshing bath!

Lemongrass and eucalyptus bath bomb

Ingredients:

- 20 drops of eucalyptus essential oil
- 1 cup of water
- 2 cups of citric acid
- 20 drops of lemongrass essential oil
- 2 cups of cornstarch
- 4 cups of baking soda
- 1 cup of Epsom salt
- Witch Hazel

Instructions:

1. Take a large bowl. Add the baking soda, cornstarch, Epsom salts and citric acid to it. Ensure that they are mixed well.
2. Take a mixing bowl. Pour the water, lemongrass essential oil and eucalyptus oil into the bowl. Mix well. Ensure that the oils blend well.
3. Now, pour the oil mixture into the large bowl containing the baking soda mixture in a slow fashion. Use a mixer to blend all the ingredients in an even fashion.
4. If you find that the consistency of the mixture is too powdery and dry to your liking, spray some witch hazel over the mixture. This will ensure that the ingredients bind well. In order to ensure that the ingredients bind well, you may have to spray it at least ten times over the mixture.

5. Ensure that the mixture is free of lumps. Transfer the fine mixture to the silicone molds. With the help of your fingers, press the mixture into the molds firmly. Make sure that you pack the ingredients tightly. This is important because the tighter you pack the mixture, the easier it will be to take it out of the molds.
6. Allow them to rest for at least 24 hours. This should be sufficient time for the bombs to harden. Once they have dried completely, transfer them to airtight containers.
7. Pop a couple of bombs into your bathtub filled with warm water and enjoy a refreshing bath!

Lavender and marjoram bath bomb

Ingredients:

- 20 drops of lavender essential oil
- 4 cups of baking soda
- 2 cups of cornstarch
- 20 drops of marjoram essential oil
- 2 cups of citric acid
- 1 cup of water
- 1 cup of Epsom salt
- Witch Hazel

Instructions:

1. Take a large bowl. Add the baking soda, cornstarch, Epsom salts and citric acid to it. Ensure that they are mixed well.
2. Take a mixing bowl. Pour the water, marjoram essential oil and lavender essential oil into the bowl. Mix well. Ensure that the oils blend well.
3. Now, pour the oil mixture into the large bowl containing the baking soda mixture in a slow fashion. Use a mixer to blend all the ingredients in an even fashion.
4. If you find that the consistency of the mixture is too powdery and dry to your liking, spray some witch hazel over the mixture. This will ensure that the ingredients bind well. In order to ensure that the ingredients bind well, you may have to spray it at least ten times over the mixture.

5. Ensure that the mixture is free of lumps. Transfer the fine mixture to the silicone molds. With the help of your fingers, press the mixture into the molds firmly. Make sure that you pack the ingredients tightly. This is important because the tighter you pack the mixture, the easier it will be to take it out of the molds.

6. Allow them to rest for at least 24 hours. This should be sufficient time for the bombs to harden. Once they have dried completely, transfer them to airtight containers.

7. Pop a couple of bombs into your bathtub filled with warm water and enjoy a refreshing bath!

Orange and vanilla bath bomb

Ingredients:

- 20 drops of sweet orange essential oil
- 4 cups of baking soda
- 20 drops of vanilla essential oil
- 2 cups of citric acid
- 1 cup of water
- 2 cups of cornstarch
- 1 cup of Epsom salt
- Witch Hazel

Instructions:

1. Take a large bowl. Add the baking soda, cornstarch, Epsom salts and citric acid to it. Ensure that they are mixed well.
2. Take a mixing bowl. Pour the water, sweet orange essential oil and vanilla essential oil into the bowl. Mix well. Ensure that the oils blend well.
3. Now, pour the oil mixture into the large bowl containing the baking soda mixture in a slow fashion. Use a mixer to blend all the ingredients in an even fashion.
4. If you find that the consistency of the mixture is too powdery and dry to your liking, spray some witch hazel over the mixture. This will ensure that the ingredients bind well. In order to ensure that the ingredients bind well, you may have to spray it at least ten times over the mixture.

5. Ensure that the mixture is free of lumps. Transfer the fine mixture to the silicone molds. With the help of your fingers, press the mixture into the molds firmly. Make sure that you pack the ingredients tightly. This is important because the tighter you pack the mixture, the easier it will be to take it out of the molds.

6. Allow them to rest for at least 24 hours. This should be sufficient time for the bombs to harden. Once they have dried completely, transfer them to airtight containers.

7. Pop a couple of bombs into your bathtub filled with warm water and enjoy a refreshing bath!

Rose and milk bath bomb

Ingredients:

- 1 cup of dry milk
- 4 cups of baking soda
- 4 teaspoons of water
- 2 cups of citric acid
- 12 to 16 teaspoons of almond oil
- 80 drops of rose essential oil
- 2 cups of cornstarch
- Handful of dried rose petals
- 12 tablespoons of Epsom salt
- Witch Hazel

Instructions:

1. Take a large bowl. Add the baking soda, cornstarch, Epsom salts and citric acid to it. Ensure that they are mixed well.
2. Add the dry milk to the mixture next and mix well.
3. Take the rose petals next and add it to the baking soda mixture. Ensure that it mixes well with the remaining ingredients.
4. Take a mixing bowl. Pour the water, rose essential oil and almond oil into the bowl. Mix well. Ensure that the oils blend well.
5. Now, pour the oil mixture into the large bowl containing the baking soda mixture in a slow fashion. Use a mixer to blend all the ingredients in an even fashion.

6. If you find that the consistency of the mixture is too powdery and dry to your liking, spray some witch hazel over the mixture. This will ensure that the ingredients bind well. In order to ensure that the ingredients bind well, you may have to spray it at least ten times over the mixture.

7. Ensure that the mixture is free of lumps. Transfer the fine mixture to the silicone molds. With the help of your fingers, press the mixture into the molds firmly. Make sure that you pack the ingredients tightly. This is important because the tighter you pack the mixture, the easier it will be to take it out of the molds.

8. Allow them to rest for at least 24 hours. This should be sufficient time for the bombs to harden. Once they have dried completely, transfer them to airtight containers.

9. Pop a couple of bombs into your bathtub filled with warm water and enjoy a refreshing bath!

Peppermint bath bomb

Ingredients:

- 1 cup of baking soda
- ½ cup of cornstarch
- 1 cup of citric acid
- ½ cup of coconut oil
- 8 drops of peppermint essential oil
- 8 drops of red food coloring
- Witch Hazel

Instructions:

1. Take a large bowl. Add the baking soda, cornstarch and citric acid to it. Ensure that they are mixed well.
2. Add the red food coloring to the mixture and mix well. Ensure that the coloring gets well incorporated with the baking soda mixture.
3. Take a mixing bowl. Pour the peppermint essential oil and coconut oil into the bowl. Mix well. Ensure that the oils blend well.
4. Now, pour the oil mixture into the large bowl containing the baking soda mixture in a slow fashion. Use a mixer to blend all the ingredients in an even fashion.
5. If you find that the consistency of the mixture is too powdery and dry to your liking, spray some witch hazel over the mixture. This will ensure that the ingredients bind well. In order to ensure that the ingredients bind well, you may have to spray it at least ten times over the mixture.

6. Ensure that the mixture is free of lumps. Transfer the fine mixture to the silicone molds. With the help of your fingers, press the mixture into the molds firmly. Make sure that you pack the ingredients tightly. This is important because the tighter you pack the mixture, the easier it will be to take it out of the molds.
7. Allow them to rest for at least 24 hours. This should be sufficient time for the bombs to harden. Once they have dried completely, transfer them to airtight containers.
8. Pop a couple of bombs into your bathtub filled with warm water and enjoy a refreshing bath!

Hot Cocoa bath bombs

Ingredients:

- 2 cups of baking soda
- 1 cup of citric acid
- 4 teaspoons of organic cacao powder
- 2 tablespoons of Kaolin white clay
- 0.5 ounce of chocolate fragrance oil
- Witch hazel

For the chocolate sauce:

- ¼ cup of raw cocoa butter
- 3 teaspoons of organic cacao powder

Instructions:

1. Take a large bowl. Add the baking soda and citric acid to it. Ensure that they are mixed well.
2. Add the white clay to the mixture and mix well. Ensure that the coloring gets well incorporated with the baking soda mixture.
3. Now, add the organic cacao powder to the mixture and mix well. Make sure that it is evenly mixed with the baking soda mixture.
4. Now, take the chocolate fragrance oil and pour it over the baking soda mixture. Keep mixing till the oil mixes completely with it.
5. If you find that the consistency of the mixture is too powdery and dry to your liking, spray some witch hazel over the mixture. This will ensure that the

ingredients bind well. In order to ensure that the ingredients bind well, you may have to spray it at least three to four times over the mixture.

6. Ensure that the mixture is free of lumps. Transfer the fine mixture to the silicone molds. With the help of your fingers, press the mixture into the molds firmly. Make sure that you pack the ingredients tightly. This is important because the tighter you pack the mixture, the easier it will be to take it out of the molds.

7. Allow them to rest for at least 24 hours. This should be sufficient time for the bombs to harden.

8. As the bombs are hardening, let us get started with the preparation of chocolate sauce. Take a double broiler. Add the cocoa butter to it. Allow it to melt slowly.

9. Wait till the butter melts completely. Add the cocoa powder to the broiler at this point. Mix well to ensure that the cocoa powder and melted butter blend well. Ensure that the consistency of the sauce is not too thick or too thin. The consistency of the sauce should be similar to that of thin custard.

10. Once the bombs have hardened, remove them from the molds and arrange them neatly on a wire rack, over a greaseproof paper.

11. Pour the chocolate sauce over the bombs in an even fashion. Though the chocolate sauce will harden within minutes, it would be ideal if you let the bombs be for at least an hour.

12. At the end of one hour, transfer the bombs to airtight containers.

13. Pop a couple of bombs into your bathtub filled with warm water and enjoy a refreshing bath!

Pumpkin spice macaroon bath bomb

Ingredients:

- 1 ½ cups of baking soda
- 2 cups of cornstarch
- 1 cup of citric acid
- 10 drops of pumpkin spice oil
- 4 drops of coconut oil
- Orange food coloring
- Witch Hazel

Instructions:

1. Take a large bowl. Add the baking soda, cornstarch and citric acid to it. Ensure that they are mixed well.
2. Add the orange food coloring to the mixture and mix well. Ensure that the coloring gets well incorporated with the baking soda mixture.
3. Take a double broiler. Add the coconut oil to it. Allow it to melt slowly.
4. Wait till the oil melts completely. Add the pumpkin spice oil to the broiler at this point. Mix well to ensure that the oils blend well.
5. Now, pour the oil mixture into the large bowl containing the baking soda mixture in a slow fashion. Use a mixer to blend all the ingredients in an even fashion.
6. If you find that the consistency of the mixture is too powdery and dry to your liking, spray some witch hazel over the mixture. This will ensure that the ingredients bind well. In order to ensure that the

ingredients bind well, you may have to spray it at least ten times over the mixture.

7. Ensure that the mixture is free of lumps. Transfer the fine mixture to the silicone molds. With the help of your fingers, press the mixture into the molds firmly. Make sure that you pack the ingredients tightly. This is important because the tighter you pack the mixture, the easier it will be to take it out of the molds.

8. Allow them to rest for at least 24 hours. This should be sufficient time for the bombs to harden. Once they have dried completely, transfer them to airtight containers.

9. Pop a couple of bombs into your bathtub filled with warm water and enjoy a refreshing bath!

Relaxation bath bombs

Ingredients:

- 1 cup of baking soda
- ½ cup of cornstarch
- ½ cup of citric acid
- 2 teaspoons of olive oil
- 16 drops of lavender essential oil
- 16 drops of cedarwood essential oil
- 8 drops of Peace and Calming
- Water

Instructions:

1. Take a large bowl. Add the baking soda, cornstarch and citric acid to it. Ensure that they are mixed well.
2. Take a mixing bowl. Pour the olive oil and Peace and calming into the bowl. Mix well first. Ensure that they blend well.
3. Pour the lavender essential oil into the mixing bowl and mix well.
4. Now, take the cedarwood essential oil and add it to the olive oil mixture. Mix well. Ensure that it mixes well.
5. Now, pour the oil mixture into the large bowl containing the baking soda mixture in a slow fashion. Use a mixer to blend all the ingredients in an even fashion.
6. If you find that the consistency of the mixture is too powdery and dry to your liking, spray some water over the mixture. This will ensure that the ingredients bind

well. In order to ensure that the ingredients bind well, you may have to spray it at least ten times over the mixture.

7. Ensure that the mixture is free of lumps. Transfer the fine mixture to the silicone molds. With the help of your fingers, press the mixture into the molds firmly. Make sure that you pack the ingredients tightly. This is important because the tighter you pack the mixture, the easier it will be to take it out of the molds.

8. Allow them to rest for at least 24 hours. This should be sufficient time for the bombs to harden. Once they have dried completely, transfer them to airtight containers.

9. Pop a couple of bombs into your bathtub filled with warm water and enjoy a refreshing bath!

Grapefruit and ginger bath bomb

Ingredients:

- 2 cups of baking soda
- 1 cup of citric acid
- 4 tablespoons of Epsom salts
- 1 cup of cornstarch
- 4 tablespoons of ground ginger
- 4 tablespoons of coconut oil
- 10 to 12 teaspoons of white tea
- 40 drops of grapefruit essential oil
- Food coloring of your choice

Instructions:

1. Take a double broiler first. Take the coconut oil and add it to the broiler. Allow it to melt slowly.
2. Wait till the oil melts completely. Upon the oil melting, remove it from the broiler and keep it aside.
3. As the oil is resting, take a large bowl. Add the baking soda, citric acid, cornstarch and Epsom salt to it. Ensure that they are mixed well.
4. Add the ground ginger to the mixture and mix well.
5. Add the food coloring to the mixture and mix well. Ensure that it gets well incorporated with the mixture.
6. Take a mixing bowl. Pour the coconut oil and grapefruit essential oil into the bowl. Mix well.

7. Now, pour the oil mixture into the large bowl containing the baking soda mixture in a slow fashion. Use a mixer to blend all the ingredients in an even fashion.

8. Now, pour the white tea over the mixture. The white tea will help in binding the ingredients well. Ensure that the mixture is wet enough to be pressed firmly into the molds.

9. Ensure that the mixture is free of lumps. Transfer the fine mixture to the silicone molds. With the help of your fingers, press the mixture into the molds firmly. Make sure that you pack the ingredients tightly. This is important because the tighter you pack the mixture, the easier it will be to take it out of the molds.

10. Allow them to rest for at least 24 hours. This should be sufficient time for the bombs to harden. Once they have dried completely, transfer them to airtight containers.

11. Pop a couple of bombs into your bathtub filled with warm water and enjoy a refreshing bath!

Gold bath bombs

Ingredients:

- 3 cups of citric acid
- 6 cups of baking soda
- 0.5 ounce of orange grove fragrance oil
- 0.5 ounce of champagne fragrance oil
- 2 ounces of cocoa butter
- 3 ounces of Meadow foam oil
- King's gold mica
- Coral orange la bomb colorant
- Witch hazel
- 99% isopropyl alcohol

Instructions:

1. Take a double broiler first. Take the cocoa butter and add it to the broiler. Allow it to melt slowly.
2. Wait till the butter melts completely. Once the butter melts, add the meadow foam oil to the broiler next. Allow the butter and oil to blend well. Remove it from the broiler and keep it aside.
3. As the oil mixture is resting, take a large bowl. Add the baking soda and citric acid to it. Ensure that they are mixed well.
4. Add the oil mixture to the bowl and mix well. Ensure that there are no lumps. Use your hands to break off any.
5. Add the bomb colorant to the mixture and mix well. Ensure that it gets well incorporated with the mixture. Ensure that the mixture is evenly colored.

6. Take a mixing bowl. Pour the Champagne fragrance oil and orange grove fragrance oil into the bowl. Mix well.

7. Now, pour the oil mixture into the large bowl containing the baking soda mixture in a slow fashion. Use a mixer to blend all the ingredients in an even fashion.

8. If you find that the consistency of the mixture is too powdery and dry to your liking, spray some witch hazel over the mixture. This will ensure that the ingredients bind well. In order to ensure that the ingredients bind well, you may have to spray it at least ten times over the mixture.

9. Ensure that the mixture is free of lumps. Transfer the fine mixture to the silicone molds. With the help of your fingers, press the mixture into the molds firmly. Make sure that you pack the ingredients tightly. This is important because the tighter you pack the mixture, the easier it will be to take it out of the molds.

10. Allow them to rest for at least 24 hours. This should be sufficient time for the bombs to harden. Once they have dried completely, arrange them neatly on a large plate.

11. Take a large bowl. Add the King's gold mica to it.

12. Take the alcohol and spray some over each bath bomb. Make sure that you don't spray too much.

13. Now, gently roll each bath bomb into the gold mica. Ensure that the bomb is completely covered with the gold mica. Use your fingers to brush off any excess mica.

14. Now, transfer each of the bath bombs back to their molds. Before you transfer the bombs to their

molds, you may want to wash the molds once and dry them.

15. Allow the bath bombs to be stored in the molds.
16. Pop a couple of bombs into your bathtub filled with warm water and enjoy a refreshing bath!

Lavender and Clay Mondo bath bombs

Ingredients:

- 2 ounces of Shea butter
- 6 cups of baking soda
- 3 teaspoons of pink Brazilian clay
- 3 cups of citric acid
- 0.4 ounce of lavender essential oil
- 3 teaspoons of Purple Brazilian clay
- Witch Hazel
- Lavender buds

Instructions:

1. Take a double broiler first. Take the Shea butter and add it to the broiler. Allow it to melt slowly.
2. Once the butter has melted completely, remove it from the broiler and keep it aside.
3. Now, take a large bowl. Add the baking soda and citric acid to it. Ensure that they are mixed well. Make sure that there are no lumps in the mixture. If you find any, try breaking them off with the help of your hand.
4. Now, pour the melted Shea butter over the baking soda mixture. Use your hands to mix the ingredients in an even fashion.
5. Take the lavender essential oil next and add it to the baking soda mixture. Mix well again to ensure that the oil is incorporated in an even fashion.

6. Divide this mixture among three bowls. Add the pink Brazilian clay to the first bowl and mix well. Ensure that the mixture is evenly colored.
7. Add the Purple Brazilian clay to the second bowl and mix well to ensure that it is evenly colored.
8. If you find that the consistency of the mixture is too powdery and dry to your liking, spray some witch hazel over the mixture. This will ensure that the ingredients bind well. In order to ensure that the ingredients bind well, you may have to spray it at least ten times over the mixture.
9. Ensure that the mixture is free of lumps. Once it is good enough to be shaped in the size of a bomb, place few lavender buds in each half of the molds.
10. Now, take the two halves of a mold and fill half of each mold with the white baking soda mixture.
11. Fill the remaining half of the first half with the pink Brazilian clay and the second with the purple Brazilian clay. With the help of your fingers, press the mixture into the molds firmly. Make sure that you pack the ingredients tightly. This is important because the tighter you pack the mixture, the easier it will be to take it out of the molds. You may not get it right the first time, but a little practice will get you there.
12. Repeat this step until the mixture in all the three bowls is stuffed inside the molds.
13. Allow them to rest for at least 24 hours. This should be sufficient time for the bombs to harden.
14. Pop a couple of bombs into your bathtub filled with warm water and enjoy a refreshing bath!

Conclusion

I thank you for choosing this book and hope you had a good time reading it. The main aim of this book was to educate you on the ease with which you can make bath bombs at home, without having to run to the store to buy them.

Bath bombs are great for people of any age, as they will make bath time a fun experience.

Adding in natural ingredients, and oils, can help you avail added benefits. Just make sure that these are all natural and not chemically infused.

Don't limit yourself to the recipes mentioned in this book and come up with different flavor combinations by your-self.

I hope you have a fun time preparing these bombs and enjoy gifting them to your loved ones!

Have fun!

39747517R00087

Made in the USA
Middletown, DE
24 January 2017